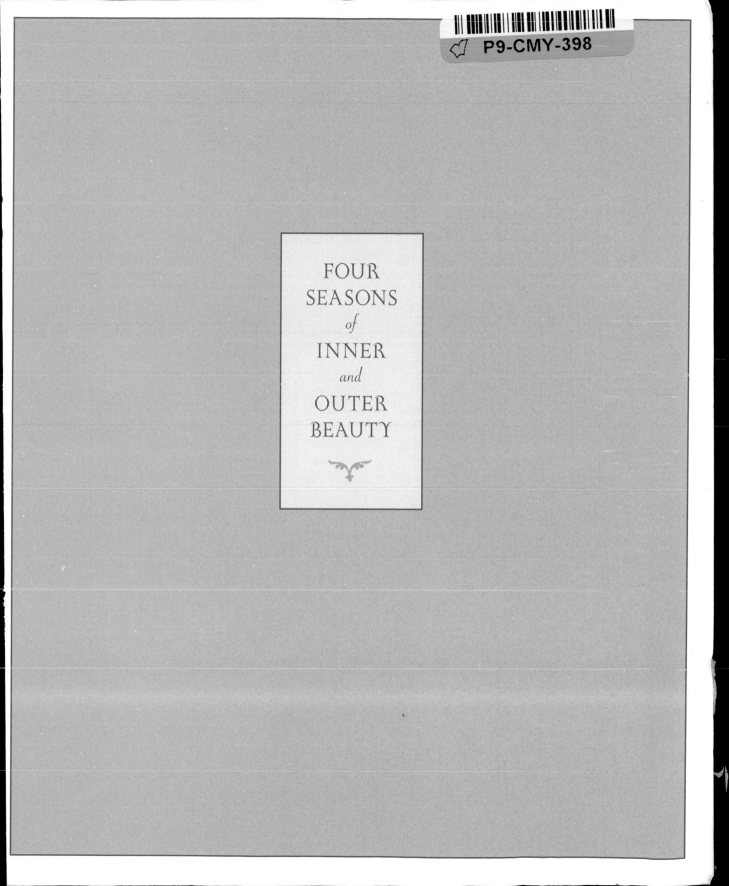

FOUR
SEASONS
of
INNER
and
OUTER
BEAUTY

B R O A D W A Y
B O O K S

·

New York

FOUR SEASONS

of

INNER

and

OUTER BEAUTY

RITUALS AND RECIPES
FOR WELL-BEING
THROUGHOUT THE YEAR

PEGGY WYNNE BORGMAN

BROADWAY

Broadway Books titles may be purchased for business or promotional use or for special sales. For information, please write to: Special Markets Department, Random House, Inc., 1540 Broadway, New York, NY 10036.

BROADWAY BOOKS and its logo, a letter B bisected on the diagonal, are trademarks of Broadway Books, a division of Random House, Inc.

Visit our website at www.broadwaybooks.com.

Library of Congress Cataloging-in-Publication Data
Borgman, Peggy, 1960–
Four seasons of inner and outer beauty : rituals and recipes for well-being throughout the year / Peggy Borgman.
        p.   cm.
Includes index.
1. Women—Health and hygiene.   2. Beauty, Personal.   I. Title.
RA778.B6675 2000
613′.04244—dc21   99-088222

FIRST EDITION

Designed by Amanda Dewey

ISBN 0-7679-0375-7

00   01   02   03   04   10   9   8   7   6   5   4   3   2   1

CONTENTS

ACKNOWLEDGMENTS

I owe a debt of gratitude to the extraordinary people who made it possible for me to write this book. A resounding thank-you to the clients of Preston Wynne. Being able to share the delight of creating well-being with you changed the course of my life.

A big thank-you to my business partner and great friend, Douglas Preston, who "loaned" me to this project for a year, shouldering assignments I otherwise would have handled. (I'm back!)

I must thank as well as our talented and knowledgeable staff at Preston Wynne. Many of the wellness practices included in this book were inspired or shaped by them. A special thanks to Edward Knightly, who generously shared his knowledge of Chinese medicine. A heartfelt thank-you for my management team, who were endlessly supportive throughout: Laura Batchelor, Paolo Preite, Margaret O'Sullivan, and Dana Barnes. I literally could not have done it without you. And every keyboard-bound author should be so lucky to have a massage therapist as gifted as Jeni De Vales.

To Judith Riven, my agent, thanks for challenging, encouraging, and teaching me. To my editors, Lauren Marino and Ann Campbell, my gratitude for making this book a reality.

I'm also grateful to my brother, David for his humor and affection, and for the support of my sister, Patricia, and her husband, Alfonso, who tried with some success to distract me by having a baby, Francesca. To my father, Ron, and his wife, Linda, for well-timed infusions of company and laughter. And thanks to my mother, Beverly, an author herself, for making books and writing such an important part of my life.

And finally, to my very patient Tino, whose ever-hopeful query "What are we going to do today?" was inevitably met with "I have to write!"—thanks for being here for me.

FOUR
SEASONS
of
INNER
and
OUTER
BEAUTY

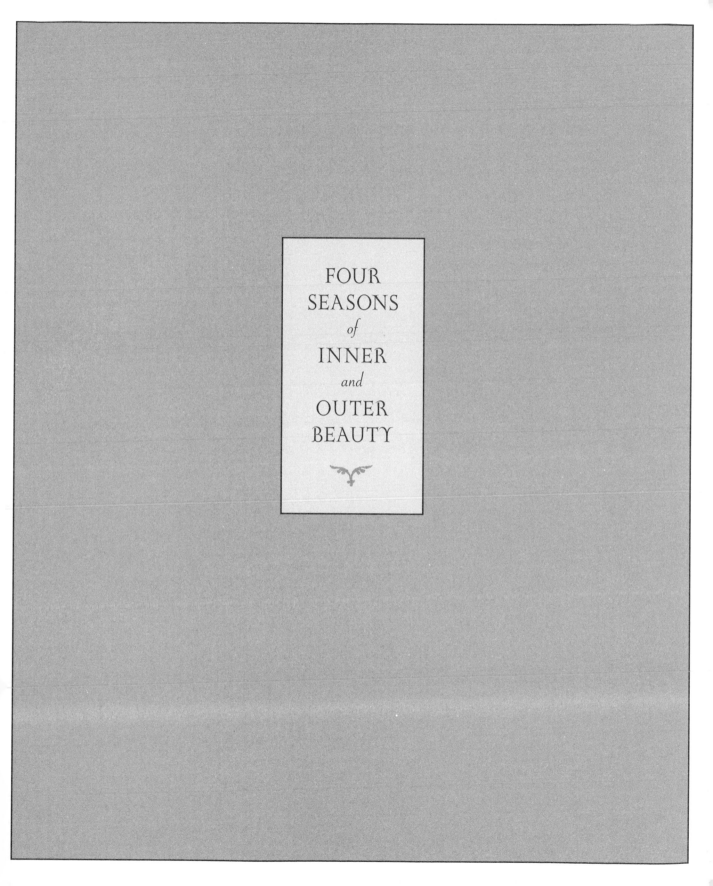

RECONNECTING
with the EARTH'S
NATURAL CYCLES

Whether you realize it or not, as you open this book today and begin to read, your response to what you find in these pages is being affected by the world around you. If it's a lovely spring morning, this book may not have your complete attention. In fact, you might be a little impatient and distracted—maybe you've already skipped ahead to find the parts that seem more "interesting." But if it's a rainy winter afternoon, you may be in a very different state of mind—you might be feeling contemplative and receptive, ready to immerse yourself fully in a book about seasonal health, beauty, and self-care.

This is a very simple example of the way the seasonal cycles influence our bodies and minds. Each season has its own distinct characteristics: Spring is a period of change and boundless creativity, while winter is a time for reflection and rest. In this book, I'll show you in much more detail how the rhythms of nature affect your mood, your health, even your appearance. More important, I'll show you how to tap into these ancient rhythms with special rituals that help you find a wellspring of beauty, contentment, and well-being.

By learning how to choose activities, foods, and sensory stimuli that are in harmony with each season's unique energy, you will feel happier and become healthier. You'll be able to quiet the chatter and noise in your mind and experience a newfound serenity. As you practice the restorative rituals in this book, your complexion and even your eyes will become more radiant. You'll find that you have more energy and more enthusiasm for your job, your friends and family, and other daily activities. Most of all, you'll come to understand that urges you may have written off as "escapist" or "self-indulgent" in the past are actually important messages that can enhance your well-being. You'll rediscover your own nurturing self, the one that's been so good at taking care of everyone else, and regain your natural healing powers.

SEASONAL CYCLES AND EVERYDAY LIFE

Each season of the year brings with it unique sensations and influences us with a distinctive tempo and energy. Although you may not realize it, your body and mind are naturally attuned to an eternal cycle of growth, ripening, harvest, and rest. With the arrival of spring, you feel renewed and eager to make a fresh start. When the summer sun shines, you grow more gregarious and lighthearted. When autumn comes, you rededicate yourself to work and get satisfaction from seeing the fruits of your labor. And when the blue silences of winter descend, you may feel quiet and prefer more solitary pursuits.

These shifting moods are part of an ancient instinct that once guided our ancestors' behavior throughout the year. When we were completely at the mercy of the natural world, our very survival depended on the ability of our mind and body to adapt to seasonal changes.

In the past, it was easier to recognize appropriate seasonal activities. If you didn't store food in the autumn, for example, you wouldn't have anything to eat during the winter. If you didn't conserve your energy and reduce your activity during the coldest months, you might burn critical body fat or run out of supplies prematurely. These days, with our around-the-clock, year-round work lifestyle, we have to force ourselves to play—but it used to be an instinctive response to summer, the season of joy and plenty. Similarly, our five senses enabled us to tune in to the subtle vibrations of the world around us and receive cues that were essential to our well-being. The smell of the air as the first storm of winter approached or the particular color of turning leaves carried both sensations and valuable information about our environment. The body and mind worked together as a seamless whole, translating this sensory language into seasonally appropriate behaviors, wisdom that enabled us to thrive.

Fortunately, our seasonal cycles haven't disappeared, they've just gone underground for a while. Without our knowing it, our bodies and minds are still reacting to the energetic shifts that occur throughout the year—shifts that can become the root of poor health, stress, and beauty battles if we try to overlook them.

The seasonal transitions are particularly challenging. Though summer continues the growth and momentum of spring, autumn heralds the end of this cycle and the beginning of decay and dormancy. Fall sets the tone for the stillness and repose of winter, but the return of spring, with all its growth and change, can be as traumatic as it is joyous. A body and mind that aren't unified and whole can be undone by these subtle seasonal changes. We may find ourselves adversely affected by the very natural cycles that once supported us.

Not anymore! As we explore the unique energies of each season, I will help you to understand the relationship between your emotional and physical state and the cycles of the natural world. The recipes and rituals included here will help bring you back into balance through appropriate seasonal activities, nutrition, exercise, and self-care. You'll soon be able to anticipate changes in yourself and others and understand behaviors and moods that might have been baffling or frustrating in the past. But first we have to take a look at how our modern lifestyles have caused us to depart from our ancient cycles.

OUR FORGOTTEN NATURAL RHYTHMS

Throughout the twentieth century and particularly over the past few decades, the natural world has come to occupy a smaller and smaller space in our lives. In fact, being "seasonless" gives us a sense of mastery over our lives. We've become experts at using technology to increase our amount of daily activity, the velocity at which we move, and the frequency with which we communicate and engage in commerce.

We maintain the same level of activity year-round, waking up at six A.M. to head to work in the pitch black of winter and using air-conditioning to fend off the lazy summer heat. Electricity allows us to ignore our bodies' natural sleep cycles as we pull all-nighters at the office or begin our evening's activities after children are put to bed. Stimulated by caffeine, our mind rattles on beyond the point at which it must rest. Any empty minute that remains can be spent in twenty-four-hour chat rooms or shopping on the Internet. We have become round-the-clock, round-the-year beings, while stress and frustration overtake us. To most of us, rest is merely an absence of activity. It is often considered a nec-essary evil. After all, Americans created the Puritan work ethic—not work for survival, but work for work's sake. And sleep? It's almost considered a luxury.

Most of us are unaware that our bodies and minds are actually designed to per-form different activities well at different times during the day; we are more men-tally alert at some times and more physically coordinated at others. Ignoring our bodies' natural cycles and subtle messages produces a pattern directly responsible for creating stress. That's because stress is not always the result of the difficulty of events in our lives but of the sheer volume of information and events we try to process. Our brains have not changed significantly in the last fifty thousand years, but the amount of information we try to pack into them has.

Obviously, stress is nothing new. Humans are perfectly designed to withstand short periods of intense stress. The survival response of the Body-Mind is activated when necessary to enable us to overcome life-threatening situations. Our heart rate accelerates, pumping blood to our muscles, enabling us better to fight or flee. Powerful hormones such as adrenaline circulate, stimulating a potentially life-saving burst of energy.

This system would work well if our fear response were triggered only by situations that were truly life-threatening—for most of us, they don't happen that often. However, many of us live in a state of chronic "stress-fear" that results from the demands placed on us by our jobs, our personal relationships, and our own goals and expectations. Our bodies continually attempt to respond to the stress and we begin to feel run-down and exhausted. And if your diet contains over-stimulating refined sugar or caffeine, your adrenal glands will be taxed even further. Stress-fear grinds constantly at us, wearing out our bodies and making us vulnerable to a host of diseases and disorders.

Many of the rituals in this book are designed to release you from the vicious circle created by your attachment to constant activity and its by-product, stress. Stress is not something that just happens to you, it's something you choose. A good resolution to make prior to exploring the rituals in this book is to stop rewarding yourself for being constantly on the go. This is not a skill worth mastering. It's one thing if you really enjoy working sixty hours a week and managing a household to boot. It's another thing if you're just proud of surviving it. Be proud of shortening your work week instead. Be proud of finding ways to say no to excessive demands on your time and energy and ensure that you have the ability to rest and recharge. You may be able to "train" yourself to sleep less, but it will create an imbalance that affects far more than just your physical and mental performance. On a soul level, sleep deprivation steals our richest period of dream time.

OUR NEED FOR
SELF-CARE

Self-care is the process of taking command of your own well-being. By doing so, you learn to heal yourself. "Healing" is not something that happens only when we are sick; it's a dynamic process of constant renewal and replenishment. The best time to heal ourselves is *before* we are stressed, exhausted, burned out, or ill. And self-care is preventive medicine at its best.

Self-care means, above all, taking the same amount of time and energy that you spend caring for others and devoting it to caring for yourself. You must learn to lavish attention on your own mind and body, making your health and well-being a priority. But self-care is not just a survival technique. If treated merely as scheduled maintenance for an overtaxed body and mind, it may simply enable us to tolerate the intolerable a little longer. Rather than relying on a monthly massage or quick-fix day at the spa to banish stress, you must incorporate both the philosophy and practice of self-care into your life on an everyday level. The seasonal self-care rituals I share with you in this book are designed to take you to a level well beyond temporary stress relief. They can and should be used repeatedly and frequently.

During the fifteen years that I've directed my spa, I've collected treatments and products from around the world, drawing on the European spa tradition as well as the Eastern healing arts. We've also discovered that modern technology has provided us with some wonderful new tools. We don't jump on the bandwagon each time a new beauty gadget is introduced; it must make sense in the context of our approach to well-being. But this blend of innovation and ancient tradition has enabled us to design a truly extraordinary menu of treatments that forms the basis for this book.

We use detoxifying seaweeds from the Brittany coast of France and aromatic essential oils from India in treatments based on ancient Ayurvedic principles. Our body therapists can provide everything from Swedish bodywork to lymphatic or

Shiatsu massage. We offer warm-stone therapy, a treatment that originated in the American Southwest, and Lomi Lomi, the traditional bodywork of the Hawaiian Islands. Many of the body-care products we recommend are made with wild herbs gathered in northern California. We also offer microdermabrasion, a high-tech facial exfoliation treatment that utilizes a controlled blast of mineral crystal to smooth and refine the skin, and antioxidant facial treatments to counteract the effects of environmental damage.

From this diverse palette we create a customized program, called a Personal Path, for our visitors. The Path is designed to usher you through seasonal or life transitions by creating a new model for your well-being. In addition to receiving a program of wonderful spa treatments designed for your specific needs, you learn how to practice self-care on a regular basis. You can attend yoga classes or consult with a nutritional counselor who designs an eating plan for your metabolic type. Seasonal workshops educate you about energetic changes that are affecting you and everyone in your life. As you spend time with us, you meet other people that are committed to increasing their well-being. And as you begin to share the benefits of taking care of yourself with your family, friends, and coworkers, you realize that self-care isn't selfish at all.

Self-care can be as simple as making a choice for well-being when unhealthy habits beckon—getting that extra hour of sleep or skipping the double mocha after lunch. Self-care can also mean doing something as elaborate as going to a spa for a week. As delightful as it is, and as much benefit as you derive from being immersed in a healing environment, I believe that integrating seasonal wellness rituals into everyday life, year-round, is the best way to promote well-being. And as much as you might enjoy your visit to our wonderful day spa, when it comes right down to it, the most important healing experience that you can have takes place at home. Though they're often incredibly intuitive, even the best spa therapists can only point you toward true well-being. Nobody knows you better than you, and inside lies a rich store of wisdom that can guide you on your path to improved health and vitality.

My goal in writing this book is to help you discover your own Personal Path through the year. The self-care practices I share make use of seasonal energies to prevent stress, fatigue, and illness caused by activities, diet, and attitude that are at odds with the earth's natural rhythms. The first and most important step is creating an awareness of your present behavior, and deciding what your body needs and what you want to change. Then you can start with the season that's in progress and proceed from there through the rest of the year. I've created this book as a self-care almanac, a reference you can return to over and over. As you experience the rituals, you'll learn more about yourself and your own unique needs, so when you return to them each year, you'll find that they've become even more beneficial.

As you begin to use these simple rituals to realign yourself with the energies of the seasons, you'll experience a new feeling of harmony with the world around you. You may find that life seems to flow more easily, or that the things that once caused you to feel "stressed out" don't have the same effect. The feeling of being mentally overwhelmed will ease. Though at first you may be a little self-conscious about some of these practices, you may be surprised at how easily they can blend into your daily routine. You already practice rituals in your daily life, many of which serve to distract or anesthetize you if you're feeling stressed. The morning run to the coffee bar is a ritual. Watching the evening news is a ritual. Your aerobics class is a ritual, and so is shopping. This book simply presents you with new choices. Self-care ultimately becomes as natural as breathing, and I'm certain that you'll find, as so many have, that rituals of rejuvenation become much-anticipated treats.

Ultimately, self-care is about love. By nourishing yourself with this vital energy, you'll regain your natural ability to offer it generously to others. In fact, it is impossible to keep the benefits of these rituals to yourself.

YOUR SEASONAL PROGRAM *for* BEAUTY *and* WELL-BEING

Though it's easy for us to feel like strangers in the natural world, human beings are still very much part of the whole. While the rhythms of the earth have become virtually inaudible in the din of our daily lives, when we stop and listen, we still recognize them as our own. Just as our ancestors did, we instinctively create our own complementary patterns, or rituals, that enable us to chart a course through the year.

Think of the pleasure you feel when you bring out the warm, woolly sweaters after the first cold snap, or take a walk barefoot on the beach in the summertime. Even the simplest seasonal patterns create the underpinnings of our lives. Season-specific sensations—the feel of the wool sweater against our skin, the sharp green smell of fresh-cut grass, the warm golden flavor of pumpkin pie, the music of a nightingale, the sight of a late summer meadow blazing with brilliant wildflowers—these are the images and sensations that create lasting memories. Our senses don't just enable us to survive, they allow us to thrive. In fact, they are a marvelous source of healing power.

In attempting to reach a place of serenity and balance, we must make use of both the healing portal of the body—our five senses—and the healing portal of the mind. Mind-centered practices heal the whole through a conscious process, such as meditation. Body-centered practices like aromatherapy heal and balance the whole through the unconscious sensory portal.

Combining Mind-centered and Body-centered self-care practices enables you to make use of the full spectrum of your extraordinary natural healing powers. The seasonal programs in this book encourage you to develop both. For example, if you are feeling overworked and distracted by a challenging project at the office, you may not be in the right state for a conscious, mind-centered practice; by choosing sensory healing instead, it will be easier for you to relax and break through any mental resistance. You will find the Mind-centered self-care practices for each season under the Healing Arts heading and body-centered practices under Sensory Therapy.

HOW TO USE THIS BOOK

The seasonal self-care practices in this program fall into two primary families. First there are the practices and activities that create balance and well-being unconsciously, using the portal of the five senses. These we call Sensory Therapies. Throughout the year, our body's sensory focus changes; being attuned to these subtle shifts will help you experience the healing gifts of each season most fully. In the spring, our sense of vision is highlighted—the better to enjoy the wonders of the reawakening world. This emphasis continues into the summer, where it is eventually overtaken by the senses of taste and smell—the better to appreciate the bounty of the season. The sense of taste predominates into autumn, where it gives way to the sense of touch. Finally, winter's stillness emphasizes our sense of hearing. This program includes practices, or rituals, for each of the five senses, and as you will discover, the relationships between the seasons and senses are both practical and metaphoric.

The second family of activities help to heal the Body-Mind through conscious practices. While they may be enriched with elements of the Sensory Therapies, they primarily engage the mind, using its powers in a positive and health-enhancing way. We call these the Healing Arts. Healing Arts rituals include Meditation, Creating Sacred Space, Making Peace with Your Body, Nutritional Healing, and Seasonal Fitness. As you'll see, these practices, too, are deeply affected by the shifting energies of the seasons. For example, as the year comes to an end and physical energy wanes, our inner life—the life of the mind—becomes more important. Meditation, even though it is a key component of self-care year-round, is the quintessential Healing Art of winter. Your receptivity to and enjoyment of the Healing Arts and Sensory Therapies will shift with the seasons.

Each season offers an array of practices under the Healing Arts and Sensory Therapy headings. I suggest letting your instincts be your guide. Try not to pick practices simply because you think you *should* do them. Choose the activities that appeal to you or spark your imagination. Your interest in all the practices will grow naturally if you begin this way, enabling you to ultimately make self-care an effortless and enjoyable part of your life. Beware of turning these practices into a strict regimen or another obligation on your list of things to do!

As you explore the seasonal programs, you will discover both similarities and contrasts in the practices. The seasonal influence shapes and guides each wellness practice, allowing us to intensify its benefits. As the year progresses, different energies in the natural world wax and wane, causing different senses to be intensified. These energics influence our mental and emotional patterns and require a shift in Sensory Therapies. By responding appropriately and making adjustments to the Healing Arts that we practice, we achieve a uniquely seasonal state of well-being.

Depending on where you live, the seasonal cycles may be more or less pronounced. Pay attention to the natural world, not the calendar. In a subtropical climate, winter is relatively short and mild. If it's still February but conditions around you are springlike, follow the spring program. Similarly, if you live in a far northern latitude, winter will last much longer. If the days are short and the weather cold and forbidding in April, continue to follow the program for the winter. The longer a given season lasts in your area, the more intense its influence and effects and the more important it is to seek balance.

If you travel between different climates and seasons, this book will be an invaluable guide to keeping yourself healthy. Rapid changes in season are a purely artificial product of our modern age. Though recirculated air on jets has been blamed for much travel-related illness, sudden shifts in climate are terribly difficult for your mind and body to adjust to. As appealing as that trip to the islands may be in the dead of winter, if you're not prepared to help your body and mind make the transition, you stand a good chance of getting sick after you get home. Jet lag can seriously aggravate the situation. Refer to the seasonal program that best describes the climate you are in to ensure a happy, healthy return.

Throughout this book, I use the word "ritual" to denote an activity that is entered into with a specific healing intent. It may be a visualization, a skin treatment, or even a meal. A ritual may require a few supplies or it could require nothing but your imagination. At times, I'll offer some very detailed instructions and recipes for these seasonal rituals, but you'll ultimately put your own stamp on them, giving them a deeper, more personal meaning.

A cyclical or repetitive quality is one important hallmark of a ritual. Women have a special relationship with rituals thanks to our menstrual cycle. In fact, the origin of the word *ritual* is thought to be the Sanskrit word *rtu*, which means "menses." The formality or predictable nature of a ritual is part of its usefulness. By designating a time or activity as a ritual, you accord importance to something that might otherwise be mowed down by the frantic activity of everyday life. An elective activity like flower arranging can't possibly hold its own against the onslaught of the to-do list. Unless, of course, arranging flowers on Saturday morning has been designated as one of your personal rituals. What do you suppose would happen to church attendance if people just went whenever they had the time instead of on a special day of the week?

Timing, then, is a key element of practicing self-care successfully. Rituals enable you stake your claim to time for well-being. Simply saying "I'm going to take better care of myself" has never worked before, has it? How are you going to take better care of yourself without making specific changes in your daily routine? Scheduled self-care rituals are the "how." The seasonal program described in this book will help you find the time and energy to devote to your own well-being. By treating these practices not just as occasional diversions but regular rituals, you are allowing their benefits to sink deep into your being and reshape your life in a healthier fashion.

THE EASTERN APPROACH TO WELL-BEING

Spas in America have their roots in European traditions, but many contemporary American spas, including mine, have also been influenced by the Eastern wisdom traditions such as Ayurveda and Chinese medicine. While European spas do place an emphasis on internal and external well-being, it is Eastern healing arts practitioners who have expanded the definition of what problems can be treated in the spa setting. The benefits of therapeutic touch and energy work have enabled spa practitioners to offer treatments that go beyond mere feel-good relaxation. The spa industry's enthusiasm for the concept of Body-Mind wholeness would not have been possible without an infusion from the East. In addition to expanding our definition of well-being, Eastern medicine democratizes the process of *creating* well-being. It encourages the individual to heal herself rather than abdicate her health care to an "expert." Most important from the perspective of this program, it encourages the individual to see herself as part of a larger whole, which includes the natural world and its inexorable cycles. Eastern medicine emphasizes the concept of living in harmony with the seasons, which is considered essential to good health.

In both Ayurvedic and Taoist philosophy, the seasons determine appropriate conduct. Seasons are viewed as an earthly expression of fundamental universal forces, or energies. Human beings, also expressions of these energies, are thought to achieve well-being only when they align themselves with these natural cycles.

If Europe has largely focused on the physical body, Eastern wellness practitioners have focused on "subtle" body, or the nonmaterial, energetic body that is thought to exist both inside and outside of us. The concept of *chi* in Chinese thought (and *ki* in Japan) refers to the subtle life energy that animates us. Techniques such as Shiatsu massage, from Japan, use pressure on points along the body called energy meridians. By opening these energy channels and restoring the flow of ki, the person being treated is healed. This is a very similar principle to the one underlying acupuncture. *Chi* energy is one and the same as the energy that flows through the natural world, and it is profoundly affected by seasonal changes.

Ayurveda, the East Indian science whose name translates to "knowledge of life," is over five thousand years old and is at the root of many other healing traditions, including Chinese medicine. It, too, envisions the flow of energy through the body, and describes chakras, or primary energy centers, in the body that govern functions from reproduction to spiritual awareness. The chakras correspond with endocrine glands and thus, Ayurveda sees a direct connection between these energy centers and hormonal activity. The first chakra, in our lower pelvis, corresponds with the reproductive glands and is thought to be the source of our will to live; the second corresponds with our pancreas and is associated with sexual expression; the third chakra is located over our adrenal glands and relates to emotional energy; the fourth chakra, or heart chakra, sits over our thymus and is considered to be the seat of love and compassion. The fifth chakra, or throat chakra, corresponds with the thyroid glands and governs self-expression and creativity. The sixth, which corresponds with our pituitary gland, is related to our intellect intuition, while the crown chakra, over the pineal gland, is thought to be the seat of our spirituality. Chakras represent the entire array of energies in our body, from our most basic survival instinct to spiritual transcendence. They are referred to as being "open" or "closed," depending on the movement of vital energy between them, which flows upward from the base of the spine. A closed or damaged chakra is in need of healing and will often correspond with a physical health condition. As we move through the year's program, you'll be able to enjoy rituals that "tune" and balance these vital energy centers, which like everything else in the Body-Mind respond to the shifting influences of the seasons.

Everyone from the ancient Greeks to modern practitioners of holistic medicine, has drawn upon Ayurveda's amazingly rich body of wisdom. Recently, much has been made of the similarity between the teachings of Vedic science, the root of Ayurveda, and contemporary quantum physics. Vedic science provides a simple yet all-encompassing worldview and fascinating possibilities for understanding the mysteries of our universe.

The similarities between Chinese medicine and contemporary Ayurveda are strong, not surprising considering their shared roots. The fundamental principles of traditional Chinese medicine and Ayurveda derive from the special properties of the essential elements that are believed to give rise to all life. The elements do not describe only a physical substance but a quality, energy, or process. They are both literal and metaphoric.

The elements engage in an infinite cycle of continuous creation. Anything we experience, any aspect of the natural world, can be understood through this universal lens. Sounds, emotions, tastes, colors, sensations—anything that you can describe or feel—is associated with a particular element. Even something as intricate and seemingly unique as our personality can be interpreted using these principles. In this book, you'll gain an understanding of the elements, or energies, and their powerful influence over how you feel during the different seasons of the year.

In this book, I employ a simplified group of just four elements: earth, fire, air, and water, an approach that corresponds with the four seasons of the year. Using these four elements will enable you to grasp quickly the most important concepts of elements/energies as they relate to your seasonal self-care program. Air symbolizes the freshness, creativity, and change that manifests itself most strongly in spring. Fire symbolizes the blazing heat, passion, and energy we experience most intensely during the season of growth, summer. Nurturing, enfolding Earth represents the richness of season of the harvest, while the Water elements evokes the still, dreamy mood of winter's rainy days. As you grow more familiar with their properties, you will be able to see their influence everywhere!

The shifting influence of the elements is not limited just to the seasons. Through the course of the day, we pass through periods in which each element attains dominance and then gives way to another. The day begins as the year begins, with the water element of night giving way to earth's expansion and opening. As the sun rises in the sky, fire energy becomes dominant, enabling us to work hard. As evening approaches, air energy urges us to share a meal and friendly conversation, read or seek entertainment. And again, as air gives way to dreamy water, we fall asleep. Understanding the element that has the most influence at a given time of day will help you choose rituals that are most beneficial.

It is important to remember that the elements are all part of the whole, and each is as necessary as any other. We all contain differing amounts of the elemental energies, but the more evenly these energies are present, the more balanced and whole we feel. The elements themselves are like compass points on a continuum. If at a certain time we have an abundance of an elemental energy—for example, fire—if the season also is strongly charged with that energy, we may find ourselves in a state of excess. If we are deficient in one of the elements and the current season offers that energy, we can tap into it to balance ourselves.

The principles of the elements are combined with the Chinese concept of yin and yang, which describes the fundamental duality of all things. It uses opposites to describe complementary aspects of the whole, both of which are necessary for balance and harmony. Yang, associated with the "masculine" qualities of expansion, aggression, movement, light, heat, and growth, is balanced by yin, which embodies "feminine" properties like passivity, receptivity, stillness, darkness, coolness, and decay. Yang rules the seasons of spring and summer, reaching its pinnacle when fire energy is strongest. Yang energy governs activities like building, working, growing, exploring, celebration, competition, dramatic performance, and vigorous play. Yin asserts its energy in autumn and reaches its peak with the water element, in wintertime. Yin energy enhances artistic expression, contemplation, gardening, meditation, playful leisure, consensus building, nurturing, collecting, sleeping, listening, and taking care of others. Yang increases and yin decreases as winter turns to spring; yang decreases as summer mellows into autumn, bringing yin energy back to the forefront.

Ours is a very yang culture, where growth, movement, speed, and creation are highly prized. It's as if we believe that a growth cycle's upward surge will last forever, that there need be no pause, no rest, no reversal, no decay. We don't understand that decline and decay lead to new growth. The rituals in this book will help you achieve balance by honoring your disavowed yin energy. Simply pausing and resting will let you welcome yin into your life. Specific rituals, such as meditation, restore yin energy, and keep us from "burning out" in yang's intense fire.

THE BODY-MIND SCHISM

In Eastern thought, the body is regarded as a physical manifestation of elemental energies and processes. There is no distinction between the subtle and the material; they are part of a continuum of creation. In contemporary American culture, however, we tend to think of the body and mind as completely separate entities. Nowhere has this been more apparent than in Western medicine.

In America, we tend to treat our body like an uncooperative third party. We blame it for our less-than-perfect health, usually oblivious of its unbreakable connection with our psychological processes. We judge it from an imagined distance, assessing its attributes and its flaws. We mistrust it, believing it to be separate from us. This sense of separation has only been reinforced by our ever-increasing ability to surgically alter it to suit our preferences or repair massive trauma that might befall it. And we feel frustrated because, against our will, it ages, breaks down, and ultimately dies. This dis-embodied, approach, if you will, creates a state of alienation from our physical selves that is wholly unnatural and potentially harmful.

Of course, we all observe some basic mind to body connections. A stress-induced ulcer, for example, is one accepted example of the Body-Mind relationship at work. Your muscle-tension headache is easily traced to the pressure you're feeling on the job. Your anxiety before a big presentation may alter the sound of your voice. However, it's not as easy to draw such a direct connection between the fury you felt toward the driver who cut you off in morning traffic and the indigestion that bedeviled you the rest of the day. And you would probably never make the connection between your stomach pain, your road rage, and the red sweater you were wearing.

A practitioner of Ayurveda or Chinese medicine would probably view this scenario as an example of fire energy run amok. The Body-Mind connection between the "hot" emotion of anger and the "hot" color of red you were wearing would be seen as fanning the flames of the "fire" in your stomach. To restore balance, both body and mind would need to be soothed and cooled. The mind would be cooled and refreshed with meditation; the stomach could be directly treated with a heat-dispersing food such as watermelon juice. And the red sweater? Your practitioner might gently suggest that it be given to someone with a less incendiary temperament.

One of the key elements of balance, regardless of the season, is resisting the urge to rush. Hurrying is one of the most common causes of a split between our mind and body. Well-being isn't achieved by finishing a project ahead of schedule or arriving at your appointment on time after a mad dash across town. Hurrying through any activity, no matter how simple or mundane, degrades well-being by removing you from the moment. Remaining in the moment means being aware of the world around you—not just the one that you've created. Lack of awareness can manifest itself in many subtle ways, such as clumsiness, forget-fulness, and an inability to focus. But there are more serious consequences to lack of awareness; if awareness is not cultivated and restored—if our bodies and minds are not in the same place, functioning as a team—immunity declines and the body becomes vulnerable to disease and dissipation. The rituals described in the Healing Arts section of each seasonal program, especially meditation, are designed to bring you fully into the present and enhance mindfulness—the real measure of body-mind harmony.

Making Peace with Your Body

Body image is an issue that most women struggle with at one time or an-other. We've been conditioned to criticize the appearance of our bodies and com-pare them to impossible ideals that we see in magazines and in the media. We're seldom happy with our weight or proportions and are constantly striving to make ourselves appear younger, stronger, taller, and thinner. It's difficult to overestimate the sway that body image has over our sense of self-worth and how profoundly it affects our enjoyment of life.

Our spa was one of the first to address women's struggles with body image as part of our body treatment program. Rather than emphasizing dramatic inch loss or weight loss, our body therapists work to create balance and well-being. We educate our clients about the results of an unhealthy lifestyle, but we also provide support and encouragement to women who may have negative feelings about their bodies.

Many of the healing rituals in this book are designed to shine light into the dark corners of you body image and help you love your body without judgment. They're designed to encourage you to nourish, nurture, and feed your body with-out apology. All too often we withhold loving care from ourselves, using it as a prize for achieving a "better" body. I can't tell you how many times I've heard a woman say that she's going to treat herself to a massage after she loses another ten pounds.

At our spa, we believe that the woman who is "waiting" to reward herself is cheating herself out of something she deserves. Chances are, she'll reach her ideal, healthy weight sooner and with less effort if she nourishes herself during that journey with wonderful body treatments. Weight that's lost through deprivation can actually become a much larger loss. We've lost happiness, we've lost a rich and meaningful connection with our senses, and, worst of all, we've separated ourselves from our bodies.

Healing body image is not just a personal process; it requires changing an entire social compact of self-criticism that women mistake for intimacy and support. In my rituals for winter, I've included an evening for friends to enjoy together, with the express purpose of affirming each other's beauty. This wonderfully Venusian ritual is the perfect antidote to group commiseration about the state of our bodies.

In springtime, we are attuned to the season when we are "springing up and unfolding," in the words of a classic Chinese text. Creating a body image that is vigorous and vital is the goal of spring's self-care program.

Summer is the season of flowering, when the unfolding of spring reaches its luxuriant peak. The urge to take off our clothes and soak up the sun's radiance is natural and, in moderation, seasonally harmonizing. But if we're shy about showing our "imperfect" body, we tend to hide, maybe even denying ourselves the pleasure of activities and events that would connect us to the celebratory energy of summer. As part of your summer program, you'll learn to care for your body with self-massage and balneotherapy techniques that enhance detoxification, circulation, and muscle tone. I share some of the root causes of figure imbalance, giving you a fresh new perspective on weight loss and exercise. I offer a visualization exercise to empower you, inspire confidence, and help your body image to "flower."

In autumn, our body image is strengthened by embracing the spirit of the earth element, which is peaceful and contented. Your autumn body image ritual focuses on the gentle art of self-acceptance and self-nurturing.

THE HEALING SECRETS OF THE FIVE SENSES

Our five senses are the medium through which we perceive and process the natural world, and therefore our senses are one of the best ways to heal our bodies and tap into the different energies of the seasons. Many of the rituals and practices in this book are rooted in sensory therapy, which involves mindfully embracing sensations, tastes, smells, sights, and sounds that promote healing and peace of mind. It is a wonderfully simple way to purify and heal both the physical and the subtle body, restoring balance in the Body-Mind relationship.

Each of the four seasons changes our sensory focus. Because our senses are constantly working together, this doesn't mean that we perform only rituals that emphasize the sense of the season during that time of year. It simply means that there is a seasonal shift in sensory awareness, focus, and acuity that we can capitalize on in our search for Body-Mind harmony.

HEALING THROUGH VISION

Vision is probably the most powerful sense of all and plays a vital role in many self-care practices. The sense of vision is associated with the intensity and heat of the fire element. One of the reasons that most meditation practices require the eyes be closed is that it's important to "turn off" this sense in order to truly restore balance to the Body-Mind.

One form of visual therapy is the contemplation of pleasing and beautiful sights. While this sounds simplistic, it is one of the most potent healing modalities we have. If you're anxious, you'll find that you can be calmed and strengthened by contemplating a glowing fire or meditating on a candle. If you're frustrated and angry, looking at the sea or gazing up at the serene sky can be enormously soothing. If you're feeling lethargic, getting up for sunrise or watching a rushing stream can have a tonic effect.

One of the challenges we face in contemporary America is visual overstimulation. We're bombarded with images from the minute we open our eyes in the morning until we close them at night. As we've discussed, the number and speed of those images—thanks to television, film, and computers—has been steadily increasing. Think of how much simpler your great-grandmother's visual environment was, compared to yours! Our ability to create and view images has far outstripped our ability to process them.

A number of the rituals in this book will incorporate a form of contemplation, or focus. No matter what the season, experiencing the landscape is one of the most important self-care practices. But I include other rituals that are designed to work with your sense of vision in a unique but limited way—for example, they may communicate with the Body-Mind through focusing on a specific color.

Color Therapy

Think of the deep blue shadows of winter and the sensation of peace they evoke. Or the gorgeous red-orange color of a ripe summer nectarine, inviting you to dive in for a juicy bite. The vivid green of spring fills us with excitement and optimism, and the rich gold of autumn's turning leaves and burnished sunsets tells us that the year's energy is now fading and turning inward. Each of these sensations balances and stimulates us through distinct wavelengths. The colors we see each season embody the visual energy of that particular time of year.

As a result, we can use the color of the season to balance Body-Mind energies. Have you ever wondered why your "favorite" color is your favorite? When you look at something in your favorite color, it elicits an emotional response: It is pleasing to you. But why? Most likely, you are attracted to colors that help to balance the energies that are unique to your Body-Mind combination. The pleasant feeling you have when looking at your favorite shade of blue is actually a signal that your well-being has been enhanced by this visual stimulus.

The primary colors correspond with different aspects of our being, and can be used to align ourselves with our activities and practices.

Blue: *Spirit*
Yellow: *Mind*
Red: *Body*

If you are practicing meditation, for example, the color blue can help create a more spiritual energy. If you're writing a report, contemplating yellow can help focus your mental powers. And if you'd like to feel sexy, well, red lingerie exists for a very good reason.

Color therapy doesn't necessarily require special equipment, though some does exist, because the medium through which you experience color can make a difference. The color of your clothing and your environment can be altered seasonally and in response to changes in your life, including an increase in stress at work or an experience that provokes grief and lethargy, such as the loss of a loved one or a divorce. Colors as they're observed in nature are the most meaningful to our Body-Mind, but for delivering color stimulation, even colored fabric will do. Colored light is wonderful because it radiates rather than reflects, reducing distortion and sending its therapeutic wavelengths zinging into your optic nerve. Think of the purity of a stained glass window and the glorious sensation of experiencing color this way. We can even experience the energy of color by infusing water in colored glass containers and then drinking it. Each season contains a ritual that utilizes its unique color to enhance the balancing and healing effect.

HEALING THROUGH TASTE

Each season of the year has a flavor that helps attune us to its energy. Spring is associated with the pungent flavor, which heats us up, increasing our inner fire. Late summer's sweet flavor is expressed in the succulent fruits of the season, and keeping pungent flavor in our diet can continue to help us attune to the warmth of summer. By equalizing our "inner" temperature with that of the climate we're in, we remain comfortable and in balance. With the arrival of fall and increasing into winter, the naturally occurring salt once found in many of the season's dried foodstuffs help attune us to the water element that rules these cooler seasons. The bitter flavor, too, cools our system, helping us harmonize with cooler weather. These flavors don't necessarily set a theme for cooking during the seasons, but when they are incorporated into dishes, they aid in our seasonal attunement.

Not all flavors are well represented in our modern diet. The bitter flavor is important to Body-Mind balance, but it's not found in many of today's most popular foods, which are dominated by excessive amounts of the "blockbuster" tastes: sweet and salty. Bitter greens, therefore, are balancing; endive, frisée, and arugula in your salad help supply this subtle but important flavor.

It shouldn't surprise you that flavor cravings are considered to be a sign of inner imbalance. A salt craving, for example, can indicate fear. Salt has the ability to direct our energy inward and downward, a grounding we instinctively seek if we're feeling insecure and afraid. No wonder that bag of tortilla chips can feel like a security blanket! If our diet contains excessive amounts of salt, we may experience a craving for sugar, which has an ascending quality and lifts our spirits—at least for a while.

The cravings created by palate confusion can be caused by meals that contain too many different flavors, especially artificial flavors. The trend toward showy and complicated restaurant dishes has abated, and many chefs are realizing that simple, beautifully prepared food is ultimately much more satisfying. With taste therapy, you will learn how to achieve inner equilibrium by balancing flavors and preparing dishes with tastes that coincide with the energies of the seasons.

HEALING THROUGH SMELL

Ten years ago, you'd probably never heard the word *aromatherapy*. Today, Glade is offering you aromatherapeutic room fresheners. But aromatherapy is much more than just burning patchouli-scented candles and enjoying the smell of fragrant oils. These nice fragrances have real benefits for our bodies and minds. The olfactory nerves have a direct line to your hypothalamus, which controls an incredible array of vital functions as diverse as sexual response, body temperature, and hunger. Aromatherapy also acts on the limbic system, the seat of our emotions.

The sense of smell is unique among the senses because it has the ability to bypass the cognitive processes of the conscious mind and create spontaneous, pure response. Have you ever wondered why a smell can transport you back in time so powerfully, evoking memories or feelings you'd utterly forgotten? In the facial treatment room at my spa, many clients get downright sentimental over the smell of camphor, the active ingredient in the Vicks VapoRub their moms massaged into their chests when they had colds as children. And let's not forget the many songs written about the lasting power of perfume!

How does a fragrance do all this? Each fragrance is an amalgam of different molecules, hundreds of tiny chemical constituents that form the building blocks of a smell. Alcohols, esters, aldehydes, ketones, and phenols are just some of the molecular components of naturally derived plant and flower extracts. The olfactory receptors—the only nerves in your body exposed to air—have been likened to locks for which different constituent molecules act as "keys." When the right key (for example, jasmone, a constituent of the essential oil of jasmine flowers) is fitted into its unique olfactory nerve "lock," specific information is sent to the brain. Jasmine essential oil is indicated for anxiety, depression, PMS, menstrual cramps, and low sex drive.

Plant and flower essences can play an important role in seasonal attunement. Though highly purified aromatherapy extracts are very powerful, enjoying the scent of fresh whole plants in season is also extremely beneficial. Aromas are powerful cues for the Body-Mind, and because of their "direct" route to the memory and emotions can quickly help to establish seasonal balance. But it's not just such associations that make the smell of a fresh-cut lawn so delightful.

Most important are the inherent properties of the essences. All essential oils, and all smells for that matter, have a cooling (yin) or warming (yang) property. The smell of that wonderful green grass has a cooling quality, making it refreshing and invigorating to the Body-Mind. Depending on the season, we may choose essential oils to balance its dominant element—cooling smells to balance summer's fire energy, warming smells to balance winter's cool water energy. The scent of rose, which blooms in late spring and summer, exerts a cooling influence over the Body-Mind, helping to balance the fire element. A bouquet of roses on the bedside table will make it easier to sleep on a sweltering summer night. The warming quality of cinnamon essential oil can likewise be used to offset winter "blues." Similarly, if we are slow to transition into the energy of the new season, we can use scents to stimulate our Body-Mind and align ourselves with the changes. If in spring we are having difficulty escaping the sluggish influence of winter's water energy, a sometimes problematic change of direction, aromatherapy extracts can jump-start us with their energetic cues. To get ourselves into the swing of spring, we could inhale essential oil of basil, which has warming and stimulating properties.

Though much research has been done to determine the effects of specific essential oils, one of the most delightful aspects of aromatherapy is that your own biointelligence will guide you to the oils with the greatest benefit for your current Body-Mind conditions. The aromas that attract and please you are the ones that are nearly always best for you. A basic "palette" of essential oils is wonderful to keep on hand, because these conditions change with the seasons. I offer a specific aromatherapy ritual to bring you into balance with the predominant energy of each season of the year. I invite you to amend these recipes by following your nose.

An olfactory tour of your palette of oils can be helpful in choosing which oils to use for specific imbalances or specific needs. It's best to do this with your eyes closed. Set aside any oils that strike you or elicit a strong positive response. Once you've created this group, take a moment to clear your "palate." You can use the old perfumer's trick of smelling some coffee beans in between oils if your nose is getting confused or overwhelmed.

If possible, work with oils that have been tested for purity or are labeled "genuine and authentic." There is a great deal of poor quality essential oil on the market, much of which has been compromised with synthetic boosters. Pure essential oils should be packaged in blue or amber glass to protect them from breakdown due to exposure to ultraviolet light.

A good home apothecary of essential oils would include:

- Tangerine
- Geranium
- Lavender
- Lemon
- Clary sage
- Eucalyptus
- Fir
- Peppermint
- Sandalwood
- Jasmine absolute
- Neroli
- Rose absolute
- Fennel
- Chamomile
- Rosemary
- Ylang-ylang
- Tea tree

Most oils, like lavender, are not terribly expensive, and most will last for about twelve to eighteen months if you store your collection in a cool, dark place. Since essential oils are antibacterial and antifungal, they are excellent preservatives— even of themselves. There are many other essential oils to enjoy, but these are some of the most versatile and beneficial for everyday use.

Lavender is very nearly a universal essential oil, and it has the unique property of being able to "marry" together other essences. For this reason, it's used in an astounding number of perfumes and scents for both men and women. Though three different oils are typically the maximum for an effective and therapeutic blend, sometimes just a drop of lavender can make your chosen essences more harmonious.

Blending Your Essential Oils

There are a few rules of thumb for creating effective aromatherapy recipes. Essential oils can come preblended with a "carrier," or base oil, typically a vegetable- or nut-oil base. For the best results and greatest economy, blend your own.

When creating my own blends, I like to use jojoba, apricot kernel, grapeseed and/or hazelnut oil. Squalane is another good emulsifying base; squalane is a lipid found in olive oil that is very similar to the oily waxes secreted by the skin. Choose base oils that are cosmetic grade, not food grade; they've been refined more completely and will be more stable. You'll find the cosmetic grade oils in the cosmetics section of any natural food store. Be careful; most natural oils turn rancid rapidly and should always be stored in the refrigerator. Your nose will quickly alert you to an oil that has rancidified. Jojoba, a highly stable oil, is good for the face and scalp, even on individuals who are oil sensitive or prone to acne. Jojoba is very similar in composition to human sebum, the oily substance our skin secretes. This enables it to penetrate and emulsify the thick, waxy buildup in our pores, helping relieve congestion. It may sound strange to recommend an oil for unclogging pores, but jojoba oil does just that.

Each season in this book contains different aromatherapy recipes, but here are some general guidelines for the safe enjoyment of aromatherapy. Because these essences are so potent, it's important to use correct proportions and proper application techniques.

• Before using any essential oil, perform a patch test. Mix two drops of essential oil to one half teaspoon of a carrier oil and apply to the inner arm.

Reapply daily for at least three days. Redness, itching, or welts are typical signs of allergic reaction. Be patient, because an allergic reaction to essential oils will often be "delayed." Unfortunately, many people who are allergic to one essential oil will be allergic to them all.

• *Very important:* Pure essential oils should not be applied undiluted to the skin. The same precaution applies to using undiluted oils in the bath. Mixing oils with a carrier before using them in the bath helps to disperse them more evenly in the water.

• Six drops of essential oil to one tablespoon of base oil is a good proportion for a blend that will be applied directly to the skin in a treatment. Essential oils are very potent and a little bit goes a long way.

• Don't blend together more than three different essential oils at one time. More is definitely not better. Very skilled aromatherapists are able to create more complex blends because they understand the interaction of the various chemical constituents.

• Never apply essential oils to broken skin. However, a drop of lavender can be used to heal minor abrasions; insect bites, and skin irritations. Its soothing and antiseptic properties make it an excellent addition to the household first aid kit. Blended with some pure cold-pressed aloe vera gel, it is also a terrific remedy for minor burns and sunburns.

• Never ingest essential oils.

• Essential oils from the citrus family, especially bergamot, can make the skin extremely sun-sensitive and cause hyperpigmentation, or brown spots. If you are using any products that make your skin more sensitive to ultraviolet rays, such as retinoic acid (the active ingredient in Retin-A or Renova), avoid the use of bergamot on the face altogether.

• During pregnancy, you should avoid the following oils: clary sage, fennel, hyssop, juniper, marjoram, basil, bay, myrrh, rosemary, sage and thyme, St. John's wort, pennyroyal, wintergreen, tansy, cedar, peppermint, and wormwood. Many aromatherapists advise discontinuing the use of aromatherapy oils altogether during pregnancy.

Aromatherapy Techniques

There are many different ways you can make use of aromatherapy. Blending a bath oil is one of the best ways to deliver your essential oils. Warm bathwater opens the pores and creates aromatic steam, which delivers the oils more intensely than any other form of aromatherapy, even massage application. I have included a footbath ritual for both cool and warm weather.

Steam inhalation is another effective way to reap the benefits of aromatherapy. Add six to ten drops of essential oil to a bowl or sink of hot, steamy water. Inhale slowly and deeply through your nose for the best effect, and drape a towel over your head to trap the aromatic steam. This is a great precursor to a facial treatment and it's also an effective treatment for colds and sinus conditions.

Warm or cold compresses, body emollients, and simple diffusers can also be used to deliver fragrances that will enhance your well-being.

When using aromatic oils in facial care, remember to apply a barrier cream after using essential oils, because they act as powerful "carriers" that can draw other less friendly substances into the skin. These creams contain emollients with a large molecular size that create a "barrier" on the surface of the skin; they discourage the penetration of anything applied over them. Even so, a barrier cream can be lightweight and appropriate for your skin type. (See Resources for the range of protective creams we recommend.)

Never apply a foundation makeup or artificially fragranced product directly over skin that has been treated with essential oil. Sunscreens and other over-the-counter drugs can become irritating if applied after essential oils.

HEALING THROUGH HEARING

Sensory information comes in waves, and sound waves bathe us constantly, from the steady hum of a computer at work to the music you listen to. The Eastern wisdom traditions have advanced practices for healing with sound, particularly Ayurveda, which utilizes "primordial" sound to heal and balance. In fact, the seven notes of the Indian musical scale correspond to the seven chakras. These single notes are repeated in ragas, musical compositions that help align the vibration of our physical bodies with the frequencies of these energy centers. Mantras are specific sounds that are either chanted aloud or repeated silently; these sounds are known for their ability to affect the energy vibration of the subtle as well as the physical body. They are most often used in meditation, where these simple sounds are believed to be energetic expressions of great purity and power, connecting us to our source. This practice has recently been supported by scientific research showing that sound has the ability to alter our physiology, even at the cellular level. On a more superficial level, one exciting new advance in skin-care technology is an ultrasound machine that stimulates the production of collagen to reverse the breakdown of the connective tissue caused by sun damage. In other words, sound can actually help reorganize the disrupted genetic codes of damaged cells and restore youthful functioning to the skin.

In Chinese medicine, each season is associated with a particular sound made by the human voice. Spring is associated with shouting, summer with laughter, late summer with singing, autumn with weeping, and winter with groaning. The rebirth and expansion of spring takes the form of a shout. Depending on our state of balance at this tricky seasonal transition where yin gives way to yang, it may be an angry shout or one of exuberance. Summer's playful, joyous energy is expressed in laughter. Autumn signals the end of growth and the return to the gentle influence of yin. The loss and sadness that may come with the end of summer is expressed in the sound of weeping. I think of winter's groaning as the sound made by a sleeper who's reluctant to awaken in the morning.

It's important to remember that these sound/expressions—even weeping and groaning, which sound rather unpleasant, really have no inherent "good" or "bad" properties. They simply give voice to the different emotional states and different energies that all of us contain. Their absence, or their presence in excess, is a sign of imbalance. For example, a woman whose speech is interrupted frequently with nervous laughter is manifesting an imbalance, as is the person who groans and moans about nearly everything. These are examples of excess, but deficiency may pose equally serious problems for our well-being. A woman who never weeps is probably disconnected from her feminine, yin energy. A woman who feels incapable of shouting may not have access to her masculine, yang energy. This energetic estrangement may be most keenly felt during the season when that energy is at its peak. The use of the seasonal sound in your self-care program releases a vibration that "breaks up" such blockages. It also helps you move through seasonal transitions when you find yourself stuck. For example, if winter's gray silence is still shrouding your mood when spring's sun begins to shine, the Shouting Ritual will enable you to free yourself and move boldly into the season of change.

The seasonal self-care rituals in this book incorporate sound in two ways. First, there are practices using created, expressed, and audible sound, such as the sound of the season. Second, some of the seasonal meditation rituals incorporate inaudible, or "inner," sound. Just as visualization is used to exercise our inner vision and can have effects in both the subtle and physical body, inaudible sound utilizes our "subtle" hearing to affect change and healing on both subtle and physical levels. We do not need to physically hear a sound to experience its vibration, just as we don't physically need to view an image to be affected by it, or actually experience a flavor to have it stimulate a physical response. Each sense has a subtle counterpart, readily activated by our imagination.

Winter, the season of stillness, is the season in which the inner voice plays the greatest role. Summer, when yang is at its peak, is when the audible voice is at its most loud and resonant.

HEALING THROUGH TOUCH

Just as we experience sound, vision, taste, and smell in many nuanced shades, we experience touch in myriad ways. The nerve receptors in our body allow us to experience pressure, vibration, pain, temperature, and texture, including moisture. These sensations play a very important role in spa therapies and are a key part of the seasonal rituals in this book. Even pain and sensitivity can tell us a lot about what is happening in our bodies, pinpointing blockages in our energy flow and showing us where healing is needed.

We respond profoundly to subtle touch, the mingling of our energy with another's. The healing benefits of subtle touch can be self-administered as well. The benefits of therapeutic touch are not produced simply by massaging muscles and increasing circulation, though that does play a key role. Healing touch often involves changes in subtle-body energies. The sense of touch is more powerful than most of us realize. As many studies have shown, babies who are denied human touch can't survive. The amount and quality of touch in our lives has much to do with our sense of security and self-esteem. To be touched with affection or respect—a warm handshake, an embrace, an arm around our shoulder—is a fundamental human experience. And mindful touching, or healing touch, is tremendously powerful. In our increasingly automated world we experience touch less and less. Even the ability to do our shopping over the Internet means there will be less social contact with other human beings, and less opportunity to touch and be touched.

The sense of touch is highlighted during autumn, when the earth element rules. Earth is associated with nurturing and protection, two activities that often involve touch. Lack of earth energy is a widespread problem in our high-tech culture. This is because many of us spend a lot of time in our heads, thinking and communicating, behaviors associated with the air element. When air becomes dominant, it is easy for us to become literally and figuratively disconnected from the earth. Touch can help to "ground" us, enabling us to become more calm and comfortable within our physical being, quelling nervousness and anxiety. These benefits can and should be enjoyed year-round, so rituals that nourish your sense of touch play a key role in each of the seasonal programs in this book.

Therapeutic Touch

It's no surprise that touch therapy, most commonly known to us in the form of massage therapy, is experiencing a renaissance. Available in many forms, it is one of the most effective ways to promote both physical and emotional well-being. The style known as Swedish massage, developed by Per Henrick Ling in the early nineteenth century, remains the foundation for much of the bodywork done in the United States. At my spa, this classical technique is integrated with Shiatsu (Japanese pressure-point massage) and Esalen, which utilizes long, light sweeping strokes to restore energy flow through the body. Reflexology utilizes pressure to stimulate reflex points on the feet and hands, which correspond to all the organs and structures of the body, and thus provides a full-body treatment. Another popular technique is Trager, which utilizes rocking and shaking movements to facilitate muscular relaxation and release of tension.

One of the primary physiological benefits of massage is that it increases circulation, which helps ease muscular tightness. Muscular tension and tightness restrict the flow of blood to the tissues, which ultimately leads to atrophy and degeneration.

Few of us think of sore muscles, even chronic stiffness, as a serious health threat. We are often able to "work around" our bodies' pain and stiffness, which lets us forget that the problem needs to be corrected. But the pain of a sore or tight muscle is an important message. I always remind my clients that the bent and stooped bodies of many elders didn't start out that way. Neglected muscular tightness can literally reshape your body, and you won't like the results of the remodeling.

But musculoskeletal problems are not the only ones eased or healed by massage. Massage also encourages the free flow of vital energy (*ki* or *chi*) along the pathways in the body, releasing blockage that occurs as the result of injury, accumulation of toxins, and stress. In Chinese medicine, energy "meridians" are linked to organs or specific Body-Mind functions, and there are points on the body where this energy can be accessed. *Chi* may be present in unhealthy excess in certain areas and deficient in others, resulting in disease and imbalance. Massage, particularly those modalities that are classified as "energy work," is a highly effective way of freeing energy and assuring its smooth flow. Shiatsu is the Japanese form of energy work, and utilizes specific pressure points to activate the flow of *ki*.

Regular massage is a vital part of self-care. In India, daily self-massage with generous amounts of oil (a practice called *abhyanga*) is performed as a preventive health treatment. This self-treatment can range from two to fifteen minutes, depending on the time available, but the optimum time recommended is at least ten minutes. Some people find this rich, oily massage tremendously helpful for anxiety and nervous tension. In Ayurvedic medicine, new mothers are given frequent massage both pre-and postpartum, and newborns are treated as well.

For learning basic massage skills, strokes, and techniques, I recommend *The Book of Massage* by Clare Maxwell-Hudson. Its clear illustrations and step-by-step instruction guide you through some good massage, Shiatsu, and reflexology routines. Though I include instruction for self-massage in a ritual for each season, a bit of work with these excellent techniques will enable you to expand upon the benefits of these practices.

Balneotherapy

Balneotherapy, bath therapy, is one of the most ancient healing arts associated with our sense of touch. Hot water was once such a rarity that hot springs and hot pools were often considered sacred sites. Western cultures attributed healing properties to mineral and thermally heated waters, and in many countries clinics and resorts have been created around them.

Though not all of us have one at our disposal, the bathtub is one of the most potent stress-reducing tools we have. As a healing modality, baths are effective, cheap, and accessible. Aromatic baths are perhaps the best way to experience and benefit from aromatherapy. Hot water can deliver aromatherapy oils both transdermally (through the skin) as well as through inhalation. For this reason, it's important to use very small amounts of the pure oils, emulsified in a dispersing base, in your bathwater. You'll find specific bathing recipes in each seasonal program.

The properties of the water are key to the benefits of balneotherapy. For this reason, I don't recommend soaking in hot tubs or whirlpools that are heavily chlorinated. The lingering smell of chlorine on your skin even after a nice soak is an unpleasant reminder that your skin is infused with the chemical. On a purely superficial level, it is extremely drying to the skin, often to the point of irritation. Thanks to the fact that it's much less chlorinated, your very own bathtub is one of the best places to enjoy balneotherapy.

Hot water does wonders for sore muscles, stimulating blood flow to the tissue and increasing flexibility. Sore muscles are not receiving proper nourishment and not eliminating waste efficiently. Enhanced circulation can speed the removal of waste from the tissues.

Yet balneotherapy is not simply about hot water. Temperature contrast bathing utilizes both hot *and* cold water to treat the body, refreshing the nervous system, and tonifying our cardiovascular system. Temperature contrast bathing is helpful for "resetting" our internal thermostat, serving to break a pattern of either chronic coldness or an overheated state. This can be very useful during periods of seasonal excess, as in a long cold spell or a prolonged heat wave. It can also assist in seasonal transitions, when we are having difficulty shifting from one energetic influence to the next. Though the ritual for a temperature contrast shower is included in our spring program, it can be used year-round.

Balneotherapy literally puts us in touch with the water element, which governs secrets, stillness, and reflection. Quietly soaking in the bath may be the one waking moment of tranquillity we experience in our day. Even if you consider yourself a "shower person," try taking at least two baths a week. Each season contains a bathing ritual designed to align you with its particular energy.

Water is also the element that is most yin, making bathing a classical ritual of femininity. Little wonder, then, that far more women than men are drawn to the bath. The bath becomes a symbol of sensuality when shared, and yang communes with its opposite.

MEDITATION

Meditation is one of the best ways to develop awareness, quiet the mind, and restore our natural rhythms of mental activity and rest. Of course, when we don't get enough physical rest, our body ultimately shuts down and goes to sleep. But providing ourselves with adequate *mental* rest is far more challenging. The mindful rest of meditation speaks to the Body-Mind on a different level. Its purpose is to dissolve the artificial structures of thinking, restoring a state of being beyond thought that reunites us with our ability to heal and restore ourselves. It's one of the most beneficial practices for anyone seeking Body-Mind balance.

Throughout the seasons, our levels of physical and mental activity vary. Spring brings a surge of alertness and energy as the Body-Mind is reinvigorated. Summer is a period of luxuriant growth characterized by an openness and outpouring of energy. We are in harmony with the energy of autumn when we practice ease and calmness in our thoughts and activities. In winter, body and mind close down and become passive, conserving *chi* and dreaming quietly as we await rebirth. Though changes in weather may make it quite obvious how to change our behavior or dress during the different seasons, mental activity must also be modulated and adjusted for the season. Meditation is an excellent way to achieve this. A spring meditation can refresh our minds and prepare us to be alert and energetic; a summer meditation can help us discover an expansive sense of joy; meditation in the fall can help release attachment and permit change; and meditation in the winter, the most meditative of the seasons, can be deep, restorative, and profound.

There are year-round physical benefits of meditation, of course, many of which have been documented, including the reduction of high blood pressure and high cholesterol. A 1987 study showed that regular meditators (practicing Transcendental Meditation) over the age of forty saw a doctor far less often than nonmeditators and had significantly fewer hospital admissions for heart disease. They also had only half as many admissions for tumors, both benign and malignant.

Of course, meditation can initially seem like the mental equivalent of a diet—all deprivation and no fun. Sitting silently and doing nothing sounds great in principle, but it takes unusual discipline to begin practicing meditation frequently. We are deeply attached to the noise and pictures in our head, because they're our primary means of defining who we are. Dismissing the noise and pictures is not only difficult at first, but it can even be distressing. The sound and fury of our lives tells us that we're important, loved, successful, and fulfilled.

As you begin to practice meditation, work on ignoring the critical or judging voices in your head that tell you to sit up straighter or chastise you for neglecting other more important activities. Their noise is just part of the static that you will learn to tune out as you focus on the clear, quiet center that exists inside you. When we meditate, we gently maneuver these powerful distracting energies *around* our quiet place, allowing them to flow by without washing us away in their rushing current. As they run furiously past, we have the opportunity to observe them apart from ourselves.

This serene vantage point better resembles the eye of a hurricane than an isolated refuge. This quiet space is literally and figuratively our center. Going there doesn't mean abandoning the world or losing ourselves. Becoming comfortable with emptiness lets us experience who we really are, free of the clutter of the ego.

In Ayurvedic meditation, which is the basis of the Transcendental Meditation technique, the meditator sits in a relaxed posture and gently turns her attention to her breath without attempting to control it. She silently or softly repeats a mantra, usually one that was specially chosen for her by an instructor. She may also use the five "universal" monosyllabic sounds, each of them corresponding with one of the five elements, which are considered beneficial for their specific vibrational quality. *Lum* is associated with the earth element and is grounding. *Vam* balances the water element and has special benefits for women. *Ram*, associated with fire, is used to increase mental strength and acuity. *Yam* is used to enhance feelings of compassion and love; it is associated with the air element and the heart chakra. *Ham* enhances communication by helping to open the throat chakra. When her mind wanders, the meditator gently returns to the mantra without exerting effort and with complete neutrality. The return is accomplished without self-judgment and with absolute comfort and acceptance.

The beauty of all meditation practice is that the *practice* itself produces the result. There's seldom an overwhelming experience that announces you've arrived in a new state of mind. Rather, the practice of meditation is often described as a gradual unfolding or an opening, one that is different for everyone. No intellectual insight can replace what's created by our mind when it's freed of its cognitive responsibilities and allowed to return to the realm of pure awareness. In this state of perfect balance, we effortlessly embody the elements, remembering that we are one with the natural world. In such a place, we are in harmony with the rhythm of the seasons. Your mind, freed of such limitations, can fully enjoy the journey through the year—and through the seasons of your life.

VISUALIZATION

The ability of our "mind's eye" to visualize is one of the great healing tools we possess. Visualization is now used in many environments where it was previously dismissed as New Age nonsense, and even Western medicine has grudgingly accepted its seemingly inexplicable benefits in the treatment of disease. Our physical sense of sight has a subtle equivalent that can be directed through visualization exercises. Visualization is an excellent medium for seasonal attunement because we can intensify the qualities of the season in our imaginations. For example, to attune ourselves to the energy of spring, we can visualize the color green or young plants budding and springing upward. To more fully experience the energy of summer, we can fill our minds with a glowing shade of red or picture a field of sunflowers in full bloom. To immerse ourselves in the energetic embrace of autumn, we can spend a few minutes envisioning a rich tapestry of leaves in tones of brown, red, and gold. To attune ourselves to the energy of winter, we can dream up a snowy scene filled with dark blue shadows and a still black pool.

Guided visualization is one of the simplest and easiest ways to effect change. In this book, it is used to create a positive body image and inspire us to take appropriate seasonal action. But in addition to the directed, conscious process of creative visualization, we can also receive visual messages. To do so, we have to make "space" in our perceptions. Instead of always projecting ourselves into the world, as we are designed to do in the yang seasons of spring and summer, we can learn to make ourselves receptive. Autumn and winter are ideal times to open to such information. When yin is dominant, intuition and insight are heightened. Native American culture has a tradition of the "vision quest," in which the individual takes a solitary journey or undertakes a fast, searching for guidance in the form of visual images. The seasonal programs in this book include rituals inspired by such practices.

CREATING SACRED SPACE

Chances are good you don't have enough space in your life, let alone something you'd dare to call "sacred space." Sacred space isn't merely territorial space, such as "my chair" or "my desk." It refers to an area of any size that has been imbued with special meaning. Not all of us have the luxury of a "room of one's own," a place we don't have to share with anyone else. Sacred space is important, for example, in the practice of meditation. While you can meditate anywhere, your ritual is enhanced by practicing in the same place every day. You come to associate the place with the practice, and as a result, you'll settle into your meditation with less effort.

One common feature of sacred space—and a perfect tool for imbuing any space with meaning—is an altar. Shrines or altars are part of many Asian homes. A shrine or altar, in its simplest form, is a special spot where objects or images of reverence are displayed and prayer or meditation takes place. Ideally, the shrine is also a haven, a quiet retreat from worldly cares.

Whether you realize it or not, you've already created altars in your home and where you work. If you're one of millions of cubicle dwellers, you may have a collection of pictures, memorabilia, and gifts displayed somewhere in your work-space: a seashell and a photograph from your vacation, or maybe just an adver-tisement for a resort you've never been to, torn from a travel magazine. Every time you look at it, you feel refreshed, transported. Maybe there's a length of beautiful ribbon from a flower arrangement that someone sent you to thank you for a kindness. Every time you look at the wisp of silk taffeta, you remember how wonderful you felt when your generosity was acknowledged. This is the magic of talismans: They speak to us in a language of symbols, communicating directly with the soul.

Self-care rituals can be greatly enhanced by the creation of altars, or sacred spaces, that provide settings for the practices. Altars can be wistful places where we lay wishes and recollections down. They can also be subtle and personal state-ments about who we'd like to be. Like so many things in our lives, the symbolic objects and arrangement of an altar have even greater resonance and power if they are selected with intent.

The place where you do your bathing rituals deserves some special atten-tion—and intention. A sacred space devoted to purification should be designed to release worldly cares and offer sensory solace. Bathing by candlelight has become an almost stereotypical image of self-care—for good reason. Lighting has a powerful effect on your mood and the personality of a space. Yang energy is increased by brightness; yin energy is enhanced by dim, soft lighting. Candles can be used as a focus for certain types of meditation, and their flickering golden light is exceptionally soothing to the soul. Aromatherapy candles, once rare, are now available in abundance. Be sure to select those that use real plant and flower extracts, not just fragrance.

Plants are nearly always a good addition, but only if you're able to keep them healthy and lush. Fêng shui, the Chinese art of controlling energy flow within a space using the principles of the five elements, tells us that plants with rounded leaves bring a more positive and supportive energy than those with spiky or pointed leaves. Even a small nosegay of roses in your dressing area will instill feelings of beauty and confidence for the day ahead. Flowers are also the perfect way to bring the color of the season into your sacred space.

Other favorite altars in our homes include the bedside table, a windowsill, or even bookshelves and desks. A bedside table can be your altar to sound sleep, while a desk can be your altar to creativity and productivity.

When creating a sacred space, the objects that you include in your altar will often be both decorative and functional—a vase, for example, or a frame for a special photograph or piece of art. They may simply be something to look at— a hummingbird nest is one of the most remarkable tiny objects I've ever found, and only years later did I learn that the Chinese consider it good luck to have a bird's nest in the house. The power of words should not be overlooked: A fine, handsome card inscribed with a wish or intention could easily be the centerpiece of an altar. Or you might include a passage from a favorite book, a poem you find moving—or that great *New Yorker* cartoon your mother sent to you in a letter. Pictures of friends and loved ones have enormous spiritual resonance. Similarly, original art, even an amateurish scribble by your hand, has tremendous power.

The colors of each season can bring their most powerful and subtle influences to your sacred space. You might welcome the joyful season of summer with an altar in every shade of that season's color, red. Or honor the color of spring, green, by adding plants to your altar.

Altars can stagnate if the objects on them lose meaning and grow "invisible" to us. The metaphor, of course, is that the same thing has happened in our lives. Some objects have such a deep symbolism that they never do. But you can derive far more enjoyment and inspiration from your sacred space if you cleanse it, revive it, and rearrange it on a regular basis. As the seasons pass, this book will offer suggestions for refreshing the objects on your altar. These suggestions will help you align yourself with the special energetic qualities of that season and create a lovely, inspiring setting for some of the other rituals in this book.

NUTRITIONAL HEALING

The vast body of traditional practices that surround the preparation and consumption of food provides us with a rich resource of healing rituals. Every culture has rituals associated with food gathering, preparation, and eating. Nutritional Healing involves much more than eating food that's good for you. In fact, most of the world's great healing traditions teach that the *way* we eat, not just *what* we eat, dramatically influences our well-being. A variety of studies and experiments seem to confirm the idea that our *intention* toward the food and drink we put in our body can and does change its energy.

If this is true, we need to begin our exploration of nutritional healing by examining our conflicted attitudes about food. Eating has become our favorite medication for stress and low self-esteem. The side effects of "treating" these problems with food transcend issues such as obesity and eating disorders—our ancient, sacred relationship with the very stuff that nourishes us has been disrupted. There is a vicious circle of eating in America. When we are not worshipping food, we're trying to figure out ways to forget about it. Our poor bodies, along for this ride, are yanked back and forth between denial and indulgence. Similarly, when we're not obsessing over food—the distressing lack of it, the chocolaty sinfulness of it—we are eating it with virtually no awareness at all. Most of us eat in our cars, on our feet, at our desks—and always much too fast. Speed and convenience are valued over flavor and nutritional value. Unwrapping a nutrition bar promises little in the way of experiential eating. The act of eating has lost any semblance of sacredness and therefore much of its healing, restorative power.

Setting and maintaining a consistent schedule of meals is one of the most health-enhancing practices you can incorporate into your life. Your body thrives on routine—whether it's sleeping or digesting dinner. Breakfast should be a light and cleansing meal, one of the reasons many of us have little appetite for anything but fruit in the morning. The "fruit until noon" practice is terrific for those who find it hard to wake up and get moving. But if you tend to feel light-headed, headachy, and irritable after such a breakfast, you may well need to launch your day with a good helping of protein and whole grain cereal or toast. Lunch should be your largest and most varied meal. A half-conscious meal on the run will not see you through the rest of the day. Dinner should be eaten early enough to be well digested before we go to sleep; it's a good idea to allow at least three hours between dinnertime and bedtime. If not, sleep will not be as restful.

Preparation is just as important. The Chinese consider the stove to be the soul of the home. If we relegate the role of food in our lives to that of entertainment or fuel, abandoning our kitchen and our stove, we cannot experience food's soulfulness. The ritual of cooking enables us to transform everyday ingredients into sumptuous dishes, imbuing them with new form and new meaning. In Ayurveda, it is believed that food prepared with love is "charged" with loving energy, and that those who consume it will be nourished not just physically but spiritually. If you, like most busy people, are eating many of your meals in your car or in restaurants, you miss this soul-satisfying experience.

The energetic changes of the seasons have always affected the type and amount of food that was available to us—until recently. Now, thanks to human ingenuity and technology, we can consume food from any season and any country year-round. Eating food during its natural growing season in your region will help to bring your body into harmony with the ever-changing seasonal energies. When the weather is cold, foods with properties of warmth—as well as warm temperatures—are ideal. And during the summer you'll probably enjoy eating cooling foods like fruits and vegetables, that balance the "fire" of the season. There's a good reason that these particular foods are so plentiful during certain times of year. Foods with warming properties are, not coincidentally, "comfort" foods. Meats, cheeses, nuts, and grains are traditionally tissue-building foods for cold-weather consumption. They're rich, high in protein, and traditionally helped sustain us through the long winter.

At our spa, we provide nutritional consultations based on the client's individual needs. Though a number of the self-care rituals in this book include special seasonal meals and recipes, I won't give detailed instructions on diet and nutrition. Just as we do at Preston Wynne, I recommend that you have an individual consultation with a nutritional specialist to discover which foods and supplements you need. Instead, the rituals in this book focus on aspects of nutrition that have been overlooked in our zeal to reduce food to nothing but calories and grams of fat, protein, and carbohydrate. We talk about foods of the season as expressions of the energies at work during that time of year. And we discuss ways to make your relationship with food more natural and harmonious.

I have also included rituals in this book that allow you to experiment with the idea of imbuing food and drink with loving, positive energy—and to perform a "taste test" to experience the remarkable results.

SEASONAL FITNESS

Learning what your Body-Mind *enjoys* is the first step toward honoring your body and developing a fitness program that is sustainable and deeply affirming. If fitness feels only like work, it is not enhancing your overall level of well-being. Pleasure, despite what you've heard, plays a key role in creating the body that you want. Why else would physical bodies have been designed with such a capacity for enjoyment? Fitness, like good nutrition, is not meant to be painful or unpleasant. Physical activity is something a healthy person usually craves.

The Eastern approach to creating a fit body has traditionally rejected the "no pain, no gain" approach. Western fitness traditions have generally ignored the role of exercise in increasing mental and spiritual well-being, focusing instead on pushing the body to ever-greater extremes and astounding new records. Thanks to our Western bias for activity, recovery has not been given its full due as a fundamental and dynamic part of staying fit.

Interestingly, some new studies are pointing to evidence that fitness programs requiring heavy, sustained exertion—such as long-distance running—actually wear out our bodies prematurely. And not just bones and cartilage. Other tissues in the body are dissipated by extreme levels of activity, causing the body to lose strength and vitality. While moderate exercise has been shown to be good for bone density, female athletes in heavy training—such as preparation for a marathon—experience bone-tissue loss equivalent to that following menopause! The anaerobic state brought on by intense cardiovascular activity is now suspected of causing an increase in the production of free radicals, the oxidizing molecules that are thought to be responsible for cellular mutation, aging, and cancer.

One size does not fit all when it comes to diet *or* fitness. Because fitness tends to be vulnerable to fads, "breakthroughs," and quick-fix approaches, it's important to begin at the beginning: self-knowledge. Creating a fitness program that gets a gratifying result and enhances your total health and happiness is a very personal process. What works extremely well for one person will not work at all for someone else. The key to creating a sustainable fitness program is to first find things you enjoy doing and *then* determine how to get the most benefit from them.

Seasonal fitness practices are best pursued outdoors, where you can absorb and experience the energy of the season. It's also an important way to absorb vitamin D: If you spend your workday inside, you need to make sure you do get some exposure to the sun. I'm always amazed to find the treadmills at my local fitness center full on a splendid spring morning. Whenever possible, do the real thing. If you're fortunate enough to live somewhere that's bike friendly, a half hour on a stationary bike and a thirty-minute bike ride are worlds apart. Which would you rather experience, the sensory information that washes over you during a bike ride or the cacophony of the typical health club, with its clanging weights, blaring television, stale air, and vibrating cardio machines? The colors, smells, and sensations of the natural world will have a balancing and stimulating effect on you when you exercise outside. In fact, a recent study showed that people running on a treadmill didn't experience the same endorphin "high" of people running at the same level of exertion outdoors. You will also derive greater satisfaction from actually going somewhere using your own physical power rather than remaining still while your feet pound a whirling belt.

Flexibility is one of the most important elements of fitness, especially as we age. The resurgence in popularity of yoga is very encouraging for this reason. Yoga increases strength, elongates muscles, and helps to reunite Mind and Body. As a fitness discipline, I feel that it's wonderfully harmonious with the spa approach to total self-care, and we offer classes in yoga at our wellness education center. Other Mind-Body disciplines like Chi Gong and Tai Chi keep our bodies strong and healthy while increasing our equilibrium and instilling us with confidence and serenity.

As you become more self-aware and in tune with your natural rhythms and preferences, it will be easier for you to recognize the best activities for you, and the best frequency. Different bodies and personalities have different needs. As we move through the year, I recommend exercise rituals that will help align you with the energy of the season. We address different elements of authentic fitness, including flexibility, strength, endurance, and energy, and suggest season-specific activities to help ease imbalance. As your awareness increases, you'll be able to make your existing workouts much more effective and beneficial. Best of all, you'll find that they integrate more naturally into your everyday life.

Remember, as we explored in our discussion of life's essential rhythms, activity and rest are two sides of the wellness coin. If you're exercising avidly but having to sacrifice sleep for your workout, you're not enhancing your well-being. Be sure to allow yourself enough time to rest and recover. On a day that you're not exercising, be kind to your body. Rest is not merely the absence of activity but an experience that can have great fullness and meaning. Rest should be considered a vital and respected component of your fitness program.

SEASONAL SKIN CARE

For years, the skin-care industry focused on the complexion and its appearance, ignoring the Body-Mind connection that is often at the root of problem skin. Beautiful skin is not simply external—it is a reflection of your inner well-being and balance. We see evidence of this when a pimple erupts during a particularly stressful time—or when our cheeks flush vividly when we are angry. The skin has a close and intimate relationship with nearly every major system of the body, including our immune, circulatory, lymphatic, and nervous systems. The skin regulates our temperature and protects us from the vicissitudes of the environment. It is an amazingly versatile organ, but for it to remain healthy and attractive, it needs mindful care. That often means adjusting your routine with the seasons.

Everyone's skin is unique, but that uniqueness goes well beyond the concept of "skin type," which usually addresses just whether the skin is dry or oily, or perhaps sensitive or "mature." Your skin is affected by your diet, your activity level, your environment, your age, and even your personality. The skin of a highly stressed, highly strung person will often be hypersensitive and reactive; someone who's lethargic and sedentary will frequently have skin that's sluggish or congested. The shifting energies of the seasons are remarkably visible on the skin. Excessive fire energy shows up as redness; excessive water is visible in pallid, rubbery complexions; earth is visible in congested, eruptive skin. Excessive air appears as dryness and flakiness. If your skin has any of these tendencies, the seasons in which these energies are at their peak will be the time that your skin will be most challenged. For example, the ruddy complexion with excess fire energy will be particularly vulnerable during the summer, while autumn brings the influence of earth and for many women a seasonal bout of acne.

A spa skin-care specialist is trained to seek out the root cause of skin imbalance. In our Personal Paths program at Preston Wynne, nutrition, stress relief, and other lifestyle factors are part of the "prescription" for improving the skin, not just home-care products. In each season, we'll discuss a treatment modality that your skin requires most at that particular time of year. However, just because you'll find, for example, exfoliation discussed in the spring doesn't mean that spring is the only time your skin will need this type of treatment—it's simply a time that the practice becomes more important to ensuring balance.

No seasonal skin-care program will be effective without a good daily skin-care regimen. The basic components of a home-care regimen are:

• A cleanser suited for your skin. A cleanser shouldn't strip your skin; it should be able gently to emulsify oil and makeup. It doesn't need to suds to do this, by the way. The lathering agents added to foaming cleansers don't make your skin cleaner—they just make bubbles. You need a liquid cleanser to truly get your skin clean, though ironically it will *feel* cleaner when you use a solid (bar)-type cleanser. Solids do not emulsify oil and oily makeup nearly as well as liquids. If you have any doubts, do an experiment—wipe a cotton pad soaked with toner over your face after you've washed with soap and water and note how much dirt and makeup remains even though your skin feels "squeaky clean." Soap and water can also cause the skin to become dull and dehydrated and can create heavily clogged pores around the nose.

• A mild toner. Most women find their skin is better balanced when they use nonalcoholic, nondrying toners. Think about what your tap water does to your shower enclosure—it's leaving the same residue on your face, causing tightness and irritation. But even distilled water can't do the job, because water's neutral pH is still about one thousand times more alkaline than your skin's. Restore the proper acidity with a toner. If you don't, you'll end up using more moisturizer than is necessary.

• A corrective or antiaging intensive. This may be a type of alpha hydroxy acid, retinol, vitamin C, or oxygen emulsion, chosen to address specific skin imbalances or deficiencies. These types of products go on cleansed, toned skin for maximum penetration and efficacy.

• Sun protection. Wear a 15 SPF or higher daily. Studies have proved that using a sunscreen of SPF 15 on a daily basis can actually reverse some sun damage you've already incurred. You'll find important information about sun protection in the summer rituals.

• A protective cream or gel appropriate to your level of oil-gland activity. With all the furor about oil-free products in the last ten years, you'd think oil was bad for your skin. It's a necessary component, whether you make your own or augment your skin's oil production with an emollient of some sort. Just remember to use only what's necessary to make sure that your skin feels comfortable throughout the day—no more. Overemoliating the skin causes it to slacken and lose tone, leading to a "mushy" texture. Some skins are highly eruptive and sensitive to oils, but not all oils cause even an acneic skin to break out. Jojoba oil, as we've discussed, can actually help break down waxy impactions in the pores.

The skin responds to a wide array of healing modalities and presents us with an ever-shifting mirror of our health, moods, and environmental exposure. In this book, I show how to take care of your skin from the inside out and how to ensure that your complexion looks healthy, radiant, and wonderful year-round, regardless of your age.

BEGINNING YOUR JOURNEY THROUGH THE YEAR

The invigorating upward surge of spring, the blossoming and expanding radiance of summer, the golden abundance of autumn, and the cool blue stillness of winter influence us all, and we are inextricably caught up in this natural cycle. By reuniting you with the ebb and flow of seasonal energies, the rituals of self-care in this book make life easier. You already have rituals in your daily life—sensory therapy and the healing arts are just healthier options. All you have to lose is your stress and fatigue!

As you begin your seasonal journey, remember that this program is not meant to be regimented. A great deal of its benefit derives from simply creating awareness of the influence of the natural world on your health, mood, and behaviors. This awareness becomes your guide. It is better to undertake the journey slowly, allowing your commitment to deepen as you experience the rewards of self-care. Explore the rituals first as they are described, then make them your own as you come to understand better your seasonal needs and preferences. I wish you well as you begin your personal path toward inner and outer beauty!

SPRING:

SEASON
OF
BEGINNINGS

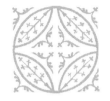

Few of us are immune to the delights of spring and to the excitement of this exquisite seasonal change. Dark skies, rain, and snow are banished; the sunshine dazzles us with its bright warmth. Our winter confinement indoors ends, and we are liberated into a world that seems new and full of promise. It often seems that each spring is unique, and the season is invented anew each time—unlike autumn, which can seem hauntingly reminiscent of seasons past. Spring offers us the opportunity to begin again, to cleanse ourselves of old attitudes, behaviors, and possessions, and set a course for a year of fulfillment and happiness.

As we long to be a part of all the newness and growth around us, we may find ourselves yearning for a new job, a new home, a new baby, or even a new relationship. We can feel confined by our winter-softened bodies and want to be sleeker, stronger, and to restore color to our skin. The natural tempo of life quickens now that the dormancy of winter has ended. Spring is associated with the energy that governs all that grows—plants, animals, and humans. It is the season of ideas, creativity, and the work of building and making, which are symbolized by the seeds we plant in the spring. "Spring fever" is not just a figment of your imagination—it's a response to the irresistible rising energy of the season, and the return of yang's influence.

Staying flexible is important during spring, as we allow our roots and branches to grow in every direction necessary. If we try to control our growth too consciously, we risk becoming unbalanced and less strong. Strength is found by allowing your growth to follow its natural course. Spontaneity, curiosity, and an open mind are important to experiencing the energy of spring fully.

Similarly, if we lack Body-Mind balance, spring can result in a quick temper and a feeling of frustration. This is yang's aggressive influence. Winter's passivity can be hard to shake off; we may want to attack our spring cleaning or a new exercise routine but find ourselves feeling heavy and lethargic, unable to act on this urge to purify our environment and ourselves. Movement and activity are essential to encouraging the flow of spring *chi*. Since everything around you is also being stimulated to grow and change, if you feel you're being left behind, you'll become frustrated and angry. You may listen to your friend describing exciting plans for the season ahead and grow irritated at her enthusiasm and energy.

Spring truly sets the stage for summer, since summer sees the flowering of the buds that emerge in spring. Imbalance now will manifest itself as imbalance in the following season. We must make sure that we clear our minds and exercise our bodies. Bathing rituals in particular help in this cleansing-and-awakening process. The self-care program that follows will help you avoid these seasonal pitfalls and remain in balance so that you can take full advantage of spring's opportunities for personal growth and change.

CLEANSING *and* BALANCING *with* HOT *and* COLD

Most of us love the sensation that follows a "good sweat," and there's a reason for it. Not only is our skin our body's largest organ, it's a principal organ of elimination. Whereas we tend to think of our skin as mere upholstery, in Chinese medicine the skin is considered the "third lung" and the "third kidney." When you perspire, you are cleansing your body—no wonder it feels great.

Sweating is one of the primary forms of detoxification and has been incorporated into cleansing and purification rituals in virtually every culture. Native American communities still use "sweats," and in Arab countries, the steam bath, or *hammam*, remains a central part of life.

While heat therapy is generally used alone in this country, some of us have used a "cold plunge" in conjunction with a steam bath, or have heard about certain hardy Scandinavians who roll in the snow after their sauna. Kneipp therapy, from Europe, includes among its many modalities the contrast of hot and cold temperatures, a process that is invigorating for the cardiovascular system right down to its tiniest capillaries.

This is an easy process to do at home, but you may need to overcome a mental block about the discomfort of cold temperatures. Once you've tried temperature contrast, you'll swear by its tonic effects, particularly for jet lag, lack of sleep, or even a hangover.

• First, take a hot shower, allowing your body temperature to rise until you see or feel a flush on the skin. Using a loofah, net sponge, or granular cleanser, vigorously exfoliate the skin. This helps remove waste that's being excreted from the pores and it also further stimulates circulation.

• Now quickly bring the temperature of your shower down to cool, making sure the cool water comes in contact with your entire body. Avoid keeping the cold water in contact with the back of your neck, a spot that is particularly vulnerable to chill.

• Now quickly bring the temperature of the shower back up, allowing your body to once again get very warm.

• Repeat this process several times, until your skin is tingling. Finish your shower with cold water. Your head should feel clear and your energy level elevated; many people feel as though they've had a couple of extra hours of sleep!

SUPPORT FOR THE CLEANSING PROCESS

Massage therapy as well as body therapies such as wraps, steam, and hydrotherapy accelerate the cleansing process and can be performed in conjunction with your "spring cleaning." They will dramatically enhance the results of a cleansing. Lymphatic drainage massage, while surprisingly gentle, is particularly helpful. Energy-balancing bodywork like polarity, Shiatsu, or Reike can also be very beneficial for normalizing your energy flow during this season of tremendous change.

THE HEALING FRAGRANCE of FLOWERS

Having fresh flowers in your living and working space is a wonderful, healthful indulgence that allows you to savor the energy of Mother Nature as she transforms water and earth into abundant blossoms and new growth. The feminine relationship with flowers is innate: The aromatic essences released by blossoms are said by aromatherapists to act primarily on our reproductive system, helping to balance the ovarian hormones.

Here are some easy ways to enjoy the benefits of floral essences and aromatics:

• Keep fresh flowers near you. A small bouquet of fragrant blossoms on your desk and on your bedside table will keep you profoundly and poetically connected to the energy of springtime. Flowers with wonderful feminine energy are tuberose, gardenia, narcissus, freesia, and orange blossoms. Roses are delightful, but be sure to choose them for fragrance instead of color. Old-fashioned garden roses are usually far more aromatic than florists' hybrids.

• Make sure that you promptly remove wilted or dead flowers. Keeping an "expired" bouquet around even a day too long will counteract the benefits you received from your fresh flowers. In Eastern thought, such visual disharmony is believed to adversely affect your well-being. Also, change the water in the vase to make sure it stays fresh.

• Treat yourself to a small vial of rose absolute, jasmine absolute, or orange blossom aromatherapy oil and wear it in place of synthetic fragrance. These three flower oils blend together beautifully to create an intoxicating perfume. A drop of lavender helps marry the flower essences.

DETOXIFYING SEAWEED BATH

The transition from winter to spring is a very significant time in Eastern medicine. Yang energy has returned and begins to expand, pushing upward like shoots of grass toward the sun. Because this represents a reversal of yin's downward, passive energy, the Body-Mind balance is in flux, confused, and vulnerable to negative emotions and illness. To protect against this, the stagnant, heavy energy that may have accumulated in us during the winter needs to be purged. Spring is one of two important periods of detoxification—the other being autumn, when yang energy begins to contract.

It's easy to dismiss detoxification as one of those New Age terms that has little meaning. But detoxification has been an important component of well-being in nearly every culture besides our own. In America, our main reference to "detoxification" is in the context of drug or alcohol abuse. The notion that the wear and tear of everyday living might create toxic conditions is still new to us but is becoming more accepted as the Body-Mind connection is documented in greater detail.

One of the most sophisticated rituals of detoxification in Western culture is found in the seawater spas of France. Seawater baths have been used in many cultures to treat disease and stress. Swimming in seawater even for a few minutes actually infuses vital minerals into the body, including sodium, potassium, magnesium, zinc, silicon, selenium, iodine, and calcium. We also know now that moving water is a tremendous source of negative ions, which impart a sense of well-being and calm.

Seaweeds selectively absorb and concentrate the mineral riches of the sea. Their potency varies dramatically depending on the region from which they're harvested. One of the most potent detoxifiers in the plant world is *Laminaria digitata*, found in the cold waters off the Brittany coast of France. Once dried, this seaweed's nutritive properties are concentrated further. It's then pulverized to remove its cellulose capsule, leaving the highly active "essence" of the plant in a very fine, rich powder. Unlike most dietary supplements, though, this one can be enjoyed either through ingestion or immersion. Minerals from seaweed or seawater can pass into the skin through osmosis during immersion or poultice treatments. If you imagine the skin as a filter, not an impermeable barrier, you can envision how this would take place. Increase the temperature of your bathwater, dilating the vessels of the skin, and the infusion of minerals will be even more rapid. This process is called, not surprisingly, "remineraliza-tion."

Laminaria seaweed attracts a remarkable array of toxins and irritants. In my work as a skin-care specialist, I used laminaria poultice masks to draw the residue of medications like Retin-A and benzoyl peroxide out of the skin when it was time to rebalance and heal after aggressive acne therapies. The area where the irritating medication had been applied would flush vividly while the mask was in place, then blanch and calm immediately after its removal. Alginates, another active element of the versatile laminaria seaweed algae, have long been used in the manufacture of paper and textiles to give flexibility and suppleness. Alginates offer the same benefit to the skin, whose outer layer, the epidermis, is actually composed of flat, dry, brittle cells—our protective "armor."

Here is a wonderful seawater bath that you can use to promote spring detox-ification and heal body imbalances. It is also an excellent way to minimize cel-lulite and rehydrate the skin. One of the finest French seaweed algae powders available for personal care is stocked by our spa store (see Resources).

• For optimum results, take a quick shower using a mild soap or gel cleanser and exfoliate yourself with a loofah *before* you take your seaweed bath. This will facilitate even greater absorption of the seaweed's active ingredients. The loofah also stimulates circulation, dilating the blood vessels in the skin and intensifying the detoxification of your entire body.

• Dissolve two heaping tablespoons of seaweed powder into warm running water to fill a shallow bath. If the water is too hot, it will reduce the active properties of the seaweed. I'd suggest adding about three to six drops of lavender essential oil to mask the pungent aroma of the Laminaria—though many people actually love the smell of the sea and find it refreshing. The lavender essential oil will intensify its detoxification and stress-relieving properties.

• Soak in your bath for at least twenty minutes. As minerals are infused directly into the skin, they will help bind water in the connective tissue, toning and firming the skin's surface. Stress literally dehydrates your skin, because your nervous system is the body's second largest consumer of mineral salts. An immersion bath is a more lasting way to regulate the skin's moisture balance than the simple application of a moisturizer.

• When you get out of the bath, pat dry minimally, leaving a residue of the sea minerals on the skin. They continue to work their magic even after the bath. Finish by applying a good hydrating body lotion—preferably one with only essential oils, not added perfume. Our Preston Wynne Spa Collection (see Resources) offers a nourishing body lotion that is free of artificial fragrance.

• Repeat this ritual at least twice a week for three to four weeks during the seasonal transition, or as often as you like. It's also very helpful if you're recovering from an injury, a cold, or the flu.

SPRING JUICE CLEANSER

Spring is an excellent time to rid the body and mind of congestion and toxin through fresh, inviting foods. The foods we are drawn to during the wintertime, what Americans have come to call "comfort foods," should begin to lose their appeal now. Winter diets traditionally include more meat and cheese, as well as stored produce like potatoes and root vegetables, which need to be cooked. In spring, fresh vegetables reappear. Eating more raw food aligns you with the profound natural urge to cleanse that comes at this time of year. The bitter and astringent quality of many of the spring greens and vegetables helps to "wake up" your Body-Mind and activate your metabolism.

If you are carrying some extra weight from winter months of reduced physical activity, a moderate cleansing or fast can be an excellent way to begin moving back toward a comfortable body weight. You will also find that nutritional cleansing lightens your mental/emotional weight and can bring about a remarkable clarity in thought. It also has a tendency to break the pattern of habitual food cravings. Keep in mind that fasts longer than one day should be approved by your health-care practitioner. If you have any health problems, consult your health-care practitioner before undertaking even a brief fast. Remember, rituals must have at their heart a healing intent. Undertaking a cleansing or fasting program with an antagonistic attitude toward your body will have a negative effect. You must listen to your body and pace yourself according to what you observe and feel.

The easiest fast to undertake is a "juice cleanse," in which you consume fresh-squeezed juices along with your Spring Cleanser. You can also cleanse with vegetable juices. Be sure to include plenty of greens and avoid high-sugar vegetables like carrots and beets. Beet greens, parsley, even blue-green algae and spirulina will satisfy your need for green. Stay away from tomato-based vegetable juice cocktails, which are full of salt.

In Chinese medicine, the organ of the body that corresponds with the season of spring is the liver. This classic cleanser recipe is considered to be one of the best for the liver; you will want to consume six to twelve glasses per day, along with copious amounts of water.

Spring Cleanser

❈

2 tablespoons fresh lemon juice (preferably organic,
Meyer lemons are wonderful if available)
1 to 2 tablespoons pure natural maple syrup (don't use honey)
A pinch of cayenne pepper
8 ounces of warm spring water or filtered water (not distilled)

I find that the juice of one small lemon will create enough for about 24 ounces of Spring Cleanser. Make sure you leave the pulp in. You'll probably be pleasantly surprised at the way the flavors blend into an appealing "hot" lemonade. Even if you don't do a fast, this cleanser is a wonderful morning tonic almost any time of year. The sour flavor is considered particularly beneficial for the liver.

EATING GREEN

The proliferation of farmer's markets across the country is a testimony to our growing interest in eating better, fresher food. A variety of spring greens arrive at this time, including baby spinach and arugula, dandelion greens, and lamb's lettuce. If you have the opportunity to buy organic greens, all the better.

The color of the season is known to artists as "sap green," a vibrant hue that's full of life. Go to your local farmer's market in search of the most pristine, most virginal, and greenest vegetables. Spring asparagus is a seasonal prize in many parts of the country and a worthy focus for a main-course salad. In Chinese medicine, the "stalk" vegetables, like asparagus and celery, are most in keeping with the upward-moving yang energy of the season. Mix arugula and frisée, which are spicy and sharp, with butter lettuce, which is more tender and sweet. The combination will give you a full range of flavor and texture. Other vegetables you might want to include are tiny beets or carrots thinned from the garden, or baby zucchini, snow peas, or fava beans.

- Blanch asparagus in boiling water for one minute, then plunge them into a bowl of ice water. Drain them, pat them dry, and lay them on your bed of beautiful greens. Whisk together a simple dressing of lemon juice, olive oil, and a dash of tamari sauce to bring out the flavor of your green vegetables. Sit down with absolutely no distractions and prepare for a little sensory tour of your salad.
- Eating slowly, first pay attention to the color of the leaves. Color is the visual sensory quality of what you are eating. What appears to be a monochromatic bowl of leaves may actually contain many beautiful shades of green, yellow, purple, and red.
- Now move your awareness to the texture of the green in your mouth. The sense of touch becomes your focus. Notice how each type of green has unique properties of sensation: the squeaky, chalky sensation of spinach leaves between your teeth; the prickliness of frisée on your palate; the fine, succulent quality of butter lettuce.
- Now direct your awareness to the smell and flavor of the leaves. Think for a moment about your breathing. Is it relaxed or hurried? Take a slow deep breath to inhale the green fragrance of your salad. Separate the tastes: the sweetness of the asparagus, the saltiness of the tamari, the sourness of

the lemon, the bitterness of the greens. Take a moment to focus on each one.

This exercise can be repeated with everything you eat, every time you eat. Bringing total awareness to the act of eating can go a long way toward healing imbalances. For those of us who feel out of control in the face of food, meals are often rushed and food is not experienced fully. This exercise will create a sensation of calmness.

Spring Dining Adventure

You deserve and need the pleasure of eating well. Nutritional healing is not only about selecting foods that enhance your well-being, but eating them in a way that super-charges their benefits for your body, mind, and spirit. With this in mind, I recommend taking yourself out to dinner, perhaps to a restaurant with outdoor seating. A change of environment can do wonders for your appetite and your rapport with food—inviting your body to experience the full benefits of eating well. More than providing a simple change of scenery, though, this ritual invites you to experience a wonderful meal as your own special guest. Too often we refer to ourselves as "just one" when we arrive at a restaurant alone.

• Choose a restaurant known for its excellent food and make a dinner reservation for one.
• Dress well, as you would for a special evening out with a companion. Do not bring reading material.

• When you're being seated, make sure you have a nice view of the dining room. Throughout your meal, make sure you look around the restaurant as confidently as you would if you were with a dinner companion.

• Accept the service as something you absolutely deserve—enjoy your server's attention and show your gratitude. This seemingly simple ritual is a rare moment in life, when you allow yourself the luxury of being served by others.

• Be sure to take your time! Notice how relaxed you feel when you're not talking and eating at the same time, or rushing to finish.

• As you eat, focus on each of your five senses in turn and explore each one fully. Concentrate on flavor and texture, savor the bouquet and feel of the wine, enjoy the subtle contrasts the chef has designed to delight the palate. And most important, don't skip any course—especially dessert.

Spring Training

As part of nature's survival plan, we are designed to weigh more in the wintertime and less in the warmer months. And as we shed our winter layers, we also become more interested in what the body underneath them looks like. You may have scaled back your fitness program during the winter, a change that can actually help to attune you seasonally. But it's important to reawaken our bodies with the return of spring.

If you have been inactive during the winter or are just beginning a fitness program, ease into it gently, steadily increasing the frequency and length of your workouts. Eastern medicine considers the kind of vigorous, intentionally stressful exercise that Americans favor to be unnatural and too hard on the body. In fact, this type of exercise is believed to cause premature aging. Furthermore, this harsh approach has a tendency to echo our attitude toward our body, when the prospect of putting on a swimsuit begins to stir up feelings of apprehension. The great American cycle of punishment and denial begins anew in the spring, when we declare war on our lumps, bumps, and bulges.

Before you begin a fast or a new diet, you need to address the state of your relationship with your body. Is it a healthy one? The body-conscious season of spring is actually the perfect time to make peace with your physical self. A new fitness program should be undertaken with respect, love, and patience. Exercise can be a powerful form of ritual healing, provided it is done mindfully and with a positive intention toward your body. This may sound simple enough, but in today's fitness culture, it is revolutionary thinking.

Ultimately, the goal of your springtime fitness program is to be in harmony with the green, young vitality of the season—to shake off the slower, heavier yin energy of winter and welcome renewed yang energy into your life. Like every other living creature, you are responding to the lengthening hours of sunlight and the stimulating colors and scents around you. Your primary fitness objectives at this time of year are:

- Get the sap flowing: Increase physical activity without hard exertion.
- Move easily, with a buoyant and loose quality.
- Get outside to absorb spring *chi*.
- Refresh and cleanse the lungs.

Here is a springtime fitness ritual that will reawaken both your body and spirit:

- Arise early and open windows and curtains to invite in light and air.
- Drink about four ounces of tepid water with a squeeze of lemon or prepare the Spring Cleanser.

• Prepare your lungs for the day by following this Ayurvedic cleansing ritual for the breath. While sitting on the floor or on a chair, put your hands gently on your abdomen. Inhale slowly through the nose, filling your lungs and feeling the expansion of the diaphragm. Now exhale sharply through the nose, drawing your stomach in with each exhalation, repeating without inhaling until you've emptied your lungs. Then take another long, slow inhalation through your nose. Breath in and out once, then repeat the cleansing breath cycle six times. Afterward, sit quietly for a minute and observe the resulting sensation. This is a good corrective ritual for nervous, shallow breathing habits.

• Begin your workout with a short visualization to attune you to the energy of spring. Stand with your knees soft, feet shoulder-width apart. Fold your arms across your chest, fingertips touching the opposite shoulders. Take three deep breaths, exhaling fully after each. Imagine yourself as a seed in the soil, your life energy curled up inside you. Surrounding you is darkness and moisture. Now imagine warmth beginning to permeate the soil. Take a deep breath and enjoy the sensation of heat. Feel it expanding your body as you fill your lungs. Exhaling, unfold your arms and slowly raise them up over your head, envisioning a bright green shoot pushing upward through the soil as it reaches toward the source of warmth. Take another breath, stretching from toes to fingertips, exhaling as you feel a breeze stirring your unfurling leaves.

• Take a brisk walk for thirty to sixty minutes. Wear a hat and sunscreen for sun protection but try not to wear very dark glasses; this is a good time of year to absorb moderate amounts of mild sunlight. Drink lots of water during your walk, but make sure it's not cold or icy. Steady, prolonged cardiovascular exercise enables you to perspire and release toxins. As we have a tendency to retain fluid during water-dominant winter, activity that moves fluid is ideal.

• As you walk, bring awareness to your movements. Don't strain, overstride, or adopt any special form such as "power walking." Keep your gait loose and relaxed.

• As you walk, affirm to yourself, "I'm enjoying this effortless movement" and "I feel alert and alive."

• Restoring or developing flexibility and resilience is important after a "long winter's rest." This simple exercise helps to loosen the back and spine. When you've finished your walk, stand with your feet shoulder-width apart, knees slightly bent. Let your arms hang freely by your sides. Inhale deeply and exhale, relaxing your arms to the fingertips. Gently swivel your upper body to the right, then to the left, allowing your arms to swing loosely around you. Don't twist your lower body; maintain the beginning stance. If totally relaxed, your hands will slap gently against your sides as your torso twists. (Envision your body as a pivot, with your arms swinging around the center and being stopped when they hit the opposite side.) Repeat this exercise for about a minute, then pause with your eyes closed and observe the sensation. The slapping of the hands against your body should provide an invigorating, energizing sensation. This type of movement and sensation is excellent for stimulating the flow of *chi*.

• At least once a week, participate in an activity that demands you be "light on your feet." This helps align you with the Air energy of spring. Tennis, ballet, basketball, ballroom dancing, and martial arts are excellent.

Remember, spring is about *newness*. So shed your faded old "skin" and treat yourself to some new workout gear. Pay attention to comfort, ease of movement, and utility, but above all have fun with it! Fresh clothing is a simple and effective source of fresh inspiration.

SPRING EXFOLIATION TREATMENT

Your skin is your body's largest organ and a participant in almost every system. Spring's transformation affects your skin as well. As we've learned, the skin's role in our respiratory system has led it to be called the "third lung." Just as you detoxify and cleanse your lungs to rid yourself of winter's residue, you should purify and renew your skin.

Exfoliation is the removal of dead skin cells. It doesn't just make your skin smoother, it actually accelerates the growth of new skin cells, brightening and clarifying your complexion. There are different types of exfoliants: mechanical and chemical. The most popular mechanical exfoliants are scrubs. Scrubs buff off dead skin cells that are loose and ready to shed. The newest mechanical exfoliation treatment in the spa world is microdermabrasion. This treatment utilizes fine mineral crystal, blasted from a special handpiece, which buffs away surface layers, smooths lines, and lightens brown spots.

Chemical exfoliants alter the skin's chemistry to dissolve or release dead skin cells. Papaya enzyme (papain) is a botanical chemical exfoliant that gently dissolves keratin protein. At our spa we recommend a gentle Fruit Enzyme Peel (see Resources) that is applied like a mask and achieves a very nice, smooth result. Nearly every clay dissolves dead skin cells. Our Clarifying Sea Mineral Mask exfoliates the skin and purges the pores (see Resources). If your skin is dry, you can prevent the drying effect of a clay by keeping the mask wet while it's on the skin—a good idea for ensuring ease of removal as well. Other chemical exfoliants include alpha hydroxy acids and retinol, a form of vitamin A. Daily use can dramatically smooth the skin, refining the appearance of fine lines and enlarged pores due to sun damage.

This simple facial-care ritual is designed to help you rid your skin of impurities and accelerate the production of new skin cells. It is a gentle exfoliation and should be done only one to two times per week, less often if your skin shows signs of excess fire, such as redness, dilated capillaries, or dermatitis. Any exfoliation is contraindicated if you have active acne eruptions or rosacea.

- Cleanse your skin with a mild, nondetergent cleanser appropriate to your skin type. Rinse well but don't use toner.
- Combine two tablespoons of warm sesame oil with a teaspoon of ground chamomile flowers (use loose chamomile tea or empty the contents of a chamomile teabag). Avoid using a microwave to heat the sesame oil, as it alters the subtle properties of the substance. Add 2 drops of sandalwood oil and 2 drops of lavender oil. A very convenient tool to warm oil for facial care or massage is a small electric coffeemaker, which you can tuck away in your "home spa" cabinet and dedicate to this purpose. The glass beaker is convenient for pouring the heated oil. Always test the temperature first.
- Apply the mixture to your skin, massaging gently with the fingertips in circular motions. Don't press down, just lightly rotate the herbs over your skin. Only briefly massage the inner cheeks, near the nose, which can easily be overstimulated. Massage the herbs into the skin for about a minute. The chamomile creates a mild grit that is much gentler than most exfoliating particles.
- Fold a cotton hand towel lengthwise and roll into a tube. Use a towel that has not been washed with fabric softener or bleach. Turning the towel end-up, run hot water into the center of the tube, thoroughly wetting the towel. Add a couple of drops of lavender and squeeze the towel a few times to ensure that the lavender saturates throughout. This trick enables you to create a nice steamy towel without scalding your hands. Unrolling the towel, let it cool for a moment to bring it to a comfortable temperature.
- Lie down and place the center of the folded towel at your chin, wrapping the ends up and across your face from both sides, leaving your nose and mouth

uncovered. Take a few deep inhalations and enjoy the aromatic properties of the lavender and sandalwood. The heat will help your skin absorb the nourishing benefits of the sesame oil. Leave the wrap on just until it begins to cool.

• Remove the wrap, wiping the mixture off your skin with the towel. Be very gentle because towels tend to be more coarse than facecloths. Rinse your face with warm water. If your skin is in the normal-to-dry range, just use toner once it's rinsed clean. If you fall into the combination-to-oily range, use a few drops of cleanser to remove the residue of the sesame oil. Follow with toner and conclude your treatment with an application of an appropriate finishing cream or gel. Our Botanical Balancer for oily skin or the excellent Moisture Creme for Sensitive Skin would be good choices following this treatment. (See Resources.)

THE SHOUTING RITUAL

Sometimes, the best way to achieve inner peace is to make some noise. In Chinese medicine, the sound that corresponds with spring is "shouting," and the weather element associated with spring is wind. This simple ritual asks you to create your own "wind," helping you give voice to your emotions in a way that is healthy and beneficial. Shouting does not necessarily mean angry shouting. Consider the energetic movement of the season, with the upswelling of yang energy pushing its way out of the earth. A shout is simply the equivalent of this upward-moving energy in the human voice.

During the spring, with so much change and activity taking place, we may find ourselves actually trying to resist growth and change because we're waterlogged with the passive yin energy of winter. Or we may be in a situation where we feel "blocked" in our attempts to bring our ideas to fruition because we are trying too hard to accomplish something a certain way and not allowing our energy to flow freely, taking its own wiser course toward a goal. The shouting ritual allows you to clear the way for positive transformation. It helps unstick the voice and free yang energy.

• Begin your shouting ritual with a minute of measured, relaxed breathing. Direct your awareness to the part of you that desires control—the part resisting the exercise. Acknowledge the resistance, take a good lungful of air, and yell for all you're worth, from the gut. A deep, nonspecific roar is best—without words. Repeat the shouts a few times.

• Afterward, return to your focused breathing for a few minutes. Observe the sensations and changes in your body. Many people will feel a sense of relief after performing this ritual, especially through the neck muscles or the sternum. You'll also notice a "buzzing" or tingling sensation as the *chi* (energy) you've stirred up pulses through your body. Observe where the energy feels strongest. The throat chakra, located at the base of the neck and close to the thyroid gland, corresponds with communication and self-expression. The shouting ritual helps relieve any congestion and can make it easier to express yourself to others—but at a somewhat lower volume!

SPRING MORNING MEDITATION

As you attempt to align yourself with the transformative growth energy of the season, use this special morning meditation ritual to clear the mind and prepare for personal growth, creativity, and enlightenment. It is best used as an early morning ritual, ideally performed between six and seven A.M. Resist the temptation to oversleep. You don't need that extra hour in bed, and by practicing this meditation regularly you will reset and balance your body clock to be able to enjoy the early morning hours of the season.

- Get out of bed and stand with your legs shoulder-width apart. Reach for the ceiling, then, exhaling, slowly roll down, vertebra by vertebra, until your hands are touching the floor. Keeping your legs straight, slowly roll back up. Then, beginning at your chest and shoulders, pat your way down your body vigorously, as if you were frisking yourself. This begins to circulate energy and wake up the entire Body-Mind. Do this pat-down for about one minute. It will help prevent you from becoming drowsy during your morning meditation.

- Find a warm, comfortable spot for your meditation. It doesn't have to be dim, but it should be quiet and peaceful. If your chosen spot faces the morning sun or a window, all the better. The easterly direction correlates with spring because spring is the "morning" of the year.

- You can sit on the floor cross-legged, with a cushion under your tailbone that tilts your lower body very slightly forward, allowing you to keep your back comfortably straight. If you like, you can use a wall or rest your back against the lower portion of a sofa or chair. You can also sit in a chair, preferably one that enables you to keep your posture aligned and gives you good support. An ergonomic office chair is actually excellent for this reason, provided you can keep it from rolling. Rest your arms on your thighs with the palms of your hands relaxed, facing upward.

- Begin by focusing on your breath. Most meditative traditions are centered on breath, which is a potent symbol of all life energy. First simply bring awareness to the breath, to the rise and fall of your chest. Breathe through your nose. Make no effort to control the speed of your breath, allowing it to slow gradually from the natural effects of relaxation.

• I don't recommend wearing a watch or keeping a clock nearby to time your meditation. You'll have a tendency to think about the time and check it too often. Just "self-time" your meditation. By using your internal clock (which knows exactly what time it is), you'll find that you can meditate for about fifteen to twenty minutes. If you meditate for sixteen minutes one day and twenty-two minutes on another day, wonderful. Meditation is a dynamic process.

• Remain motionless for at least five minutes. Don't adjust your body in any way. The only motion should be from your breath, as your chest expands and contracts.

• Now envision your breath as a glistening mist made dazzling by the rays of a glorious morning sun. Picture it surging into your body and swirling inside you; then envision this brilliant mist being released into the air as you exhale. Savor the sense of emptiness at the end of your exhalation; don't rush into your next inhalation. Quietly feel the tension, the slight vacuum, at the end of your breath, and then inhale once again, drawing in this immense, dazzling cloud of energy. Hold it as it spirals and swirls inside you, energizing your entire body.

• Now draw in a breath and envision the mist lighting up the inside of your body. Picture yourself glowing from within like a lightbulb. As you exhale, envision this effulgent cloud exiting your body in a cascade of tiny stars through your hands, your fingertips, your feet, your toes. Envision your body growing lighter and more transparent as the glowing from within becomes brighter still.

• When you next inhale and exhale, envision the glowing cloud being released through your skin, your pores. The heavenly cloud dissolves you in its brilliance, and inhaling and exhaling, you become pure light.

• To conclude the meditation, visualize the glistening cloud of light coalescing and gradually taking on form. Envision your body reappearing in its familiar material form but now transformed with tremendous energy. Move your hands and feet to reconnect to the physical experience of your body, keeping your eyes closed for a minute or so longer. Then slowly open your eyes. You should find a spring morning filled with promise.

Some good questions to ask yourself following a springtime meditation are:

Am I growing?

How am I expressing my natural creativity?

Am I resisting growth and change? How?

Am I honoring growth and change in others? How am I doing this?

• A wonderful way to top off your meditation is with a short writing ritual. Take just a moment to write down on a small piece of paper three things you would like to accomplish that day. Don't labor over this. Think of it not as a list of things to do but as three wishes.

• Your wish might be something simple, like "apologize to Susan," or something more grand, like "submit résumé for new job." Directing intention to do these things is the first step toward making them real. Carry this with you for the entire day, and at the end of the day discard it. The last thing you want is for your wishes to become stressors or "unfinished business." You may choose them again in a subsequent meditation, but it's always good to remain open to new wishes and intentions.

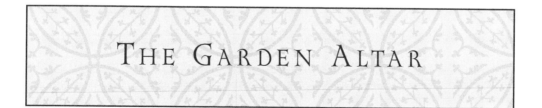

THE GARDEN ALTAR

Springtime inspires many of us to clean our homes and personal space of clutter and old possessions—spring housecleaning is a "detoxification" of the environment in which we live and work. We find ourselves purging things we may consciously or unconsciously feel are holding us back, preventing us from joining in the momentum of growth and change that characterizes the season. Even objects we were quite attached to can be seen in a different light as the rest of the world takes on a shiny new quality. The room that seemed cozy the previous fall now seems dark. Indoor air smells stale and lifeless. We throw open windows and invite the wind to scour away the odors of our quiet winter life. In the Taoist tradition, the fifth day of the fifth moon of the year is a time of purification and cleansing. Religious rites are performed at the temple or ritual hall, but lay people also clean and renew their homes and altars at this time.

Even if you don't have a yard or garden, the desire to clear away the dead undergrowth and open up an area to sow can be very strong. Getting out into a garden is one of the best activities for aligning yourself with the energy of spring. Gardening is an important part of many spiritual practices and traditions, and gardens themselves are often associated with and become holy places.

Gardens can be experienced on many levels. At its most basic, a garden is the intersection of nature's gifts and our intentions. It is a collaboration between us and our creator. Above all, gardens must be tended and worked, weeds removed and plants watered and fed, much in the same way we must tend to and nurture ourselves.

A spring garden altar is a way for you to acknowledge, honor, and enjoy all that is green, alive, and growing. An altar simply creates a visual reminder of our place in the yearly cycle and can be a focus for meditation and contemplation. The garden altar may be indoors or out. Here are some of spring's elements that you can include:

• Incorporate the brilliant green color of the season, using plants, moss, or grasses. Moss is lovely used at the base of a dish-type flower arrangement. Grasses are often overlooked in favor of more ornamental foliage, but they embody the spirit of springtime beautifully since they are some of the first new growth we see. Wheatgrass, which can be grown in a shallow container, is one of the simplest and most beautiful expressions of the color of the season.

• Fragrant flowers of the season are naturally the star of the spring altar. Grow a potful of narcissus, daffodils, or tulips from bulbs. Observing the daily progress of the flowers aligns you with spring's growth energy.

• A vessel or pretty container for water, which cleanses and nourishes the growth of spring. This can be a fountain, pool, or beautiful bowl with a flower floating in it. Make sure the water is impeccably fresh.

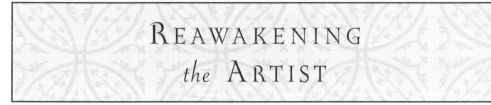

REAWAKENING *the* ARTIST

As children, art was a natural part of our lives. Expressing ourselves with paint and crayons was easy—until we grew old enough to realize that our artistic expressions could be judged. Fear of that judgment has caused many of us to lose touch with our artistic selves. Spring is an excellent time to reawaken that creative spirit or begin an artistic pursuit, especially if you've never considered yourself to be creative or artistically talented. It is the season in which we are most receptive to learning.

Sketching or painting can be a meditative way to reclaim just five minutes for yourself—while waiting for the kids to finish soccer practice, or as a way to conclude your workday when you arrive home. Making even a simple sketch is still an act of creation, one of the joys of our existence. Drawing and painting with children is another wonderful way to celebrate and optimize the creative energy of spring. Let yourself be inspired by their example. Your analytical left brain should not be part of this process. The creative, spontaneous right brain is the source of artistic urges.

• Take a small sketchbook and watercolor pen—something you can slip inside your bag—with you wherever you go. You'll find compelling subjects in the most mundane settings, and your eyes and hand will rediscover their natural artistic kinship.

• Stimulate the Body-Mind by using color. Colored pencils are clean and easy to carry, but if you want to experience color more intensely, watercolors are ideal. A favorite tool of spontaneous painters is Winsor Newton's tiny but self-contained Cotman watercolor kit, which is about the size of a cellular phone.

To help you lose your inhibitions about drawing, try this series of simple exercises:

• If you're right handed, put a piece of charcoal in your left hand; if left handed, switch to your right. Don't worry about creating a recognizable image. Place your charcoal on the pad and, without looking down at it, record the contour of a simple object, such as a vase, a book, or a shoe. Spend about twenty minutes, repeating the exercise about ten times. This helps to break eye/hand habits that prevent us from really seeing an object afresh.

• Now focus your attention only on the light/dark contrast you see. Forget about lines and outlines altogether. Without looking at the page, take the broad side of the charcoal and loosely indicate the areas of darkness and shadow you observe on and around the object. Make a half dozen of these value-contrast sketches, spending only two minutes on each one. You'll be surprised at how much more you're beginning to see now that you're not relating to the object in a linear fashion.

• Next, imagine yourself inside the object. Find its core or center. Once again, resist the temptation to look at the page until you're done with the exercise. Using rapid, "three-dimensional" circular strokes, add mass to the core, building your object up from the inside out. This will help connect you to the essence of the object rather than just its surface contours. Repeat this exercise about six times, spending no more than a couple of minutes on each one.

• Now look for the movement of the object's lines and planes. Exaggerate any "gesture" you see. If you see a shape that moves up and out, use bold directional strokes to indicate that movement. If you see roundness, carve curves into the page vigorously. This exercise is about energy. Don't worry about perspective! Think about the strength of the object's lines. Try to put that same strength into the strokes of the charcoal.

If you repeat these exercises about three times a week, you'll be surprised at how differently you'll approach drawing. You'll lose your inhibition and tendency to judge your finished product and become more attuned to the immediate experience, instead.

YOUR VISION *for* *the* YEAR AHEAD

Spring is an excellent time for a vacation—not to play but to think clearly about the year ahead and what you'd like to make of it. If at all possible, plan a short retreat to focus on your life purpose and goals. Go with a like-minded friend, or better yet, alone. Your destination can be as spartan or luxurious as you wish, but it should have minimal distractions so you can stay focused on your central purpose. There is nothing like the natural beauty of the landscape to inspire contemplation. Observing silence for long periods of time is a fundamental part of a retreat, and it can be difficult at first. Don't worry; the healing power of silence, stillness, and solitude will reveal itself to you.

There are a number of monasteries managed by religious orders that are open to the public, where personal retreats are not only welcomed but encouraged. Most of these retreats and sanctuaries are simply appointed and inexpensive. Many are in magnificent and inspiring locations, such as the New Camaldoli monastery perched high on California's Big Sur coast or the Monastery of Christ in the Desert, near Abiquiu, New Mexico. Though you are welcome to join the residents for religious services, it is usually voluntary. *Paradise Found* by Stanley Young is a beautiful guide to retreats and sanctuaries in the West and the Southwest.

Take a tool for reflection, a blank notebook and any other materials you enjoy working with such as pens or paints. Leave your laptop at home. Plan your time to include the rituals listed in this section twice a day. Here are some other ideas to make your weekend retreat restorative and relaxing:

• A brisk walk upon rising will help you clear your head for contemplation.

• Avoid any caffeine or alcohol, and cleanse your system with plenty of water. A small amount of properly prepared, good green tea can actually help clarify your thoughts and awaken insight. Jasmine pearl tea (available from the specialty Chinese tea importer or store) is one of the most exquisite. It should be prepared with hot but not boiling water. Four of the "pearls" will brew a surprisingly fragrant cup of tea.

• Listen to your body, resting or napping when you feel tired.

• If it's available, have at least one massage during your retreat.

• Rise early to enjoy the sunrise.

• Meditate once in the morning and once in the afternoon.

• Practice the drawing exercise in this section. An unfamiliar setting will make it even easier to let go of eye/hand habits. Drawing aids in contemplation.

• Reflect and write on your goals for:

Physical health
Emotional wellness
Work
Relationships
Spiritual growth

When you return from your retreat, refer to your journal frequently to renew your goals for the year. Your memories of this experience will help you remain strong, balanced, and resourceful during periods of challenge or stress. A personal retreat is a wonderful ritual to observe year after year.

SUMMER:
SEASON
OF
EXPANSION

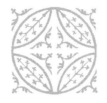

The predominant emotion of summer is joy, and everywhere you feel the expansive quality of the season's energy. The promise of spring is being fulfilled; its buds have become the abundant flowers and fruit of summer. Gardens grow lush, the days grow longer, and the evenings are suffused with light. Our *chi* is moving outward and expanding in the radiance of the summer sun. There is more movement and physical activity, though it must be moderated to prevent summer's fire from overtaking us. In the fire element, yin and yang intermingle; summer is a time when hearts open. The heart chakra should be open and ready to receive the season's gifts: joy and the warm companionship of others. Friends and family are the natural focus of our attention.

Play becomes as important as work and a long-anticipated summer vacation may become the center of our attention. Fire energy inspires communication, so this can be a productive time for activities and projects that emphasize interaction with others. At work, unless you're involved in something creative and engrossing—an exciting new project or a job that you love—you may well find yourself daydreaming at your desk or concocting excuses to leave early. Our Body-Mind instinctively knows that right now we need to be outdoors, soaking up the warmth and stimulating our brains with the full range of sunlight's wavelengths. The city dweller seeks out the park, and just the sight of other people at play expands her heart.

Creativity is also associated with the fire element, as is intuition and action. Taken together, these are the qualities necessary to bring endeavors to fruition, to "make things happen." We may find ourselves feeling unstoppable, confident, and full of energy and plans. For those of us who tend to be more doubtful or hesitant, summer is an ideal time to absorb some of this empowering go-getter energy. But we can also get out of balance if we don't modulate our activity. Fire energy is exciting and alluring, but if we get too much of it, we become overwhelmed, exhausted, and "burn out." One of the best cures for excessive heat is water, and that is indeed where many of us head during the summertime, whether it's to a lake, river, or ocean. Not surprisingly, our fire energy is at its peak from eleven A.M. to one P.M., when the sun is high. Though you may not feel like it this early in the day, it is a good time to rest and take a break.

The interpenetration of feminine yin and masculine yang during the summer ensures that this is a time when love is in the air. Summer is indeed the season of the heart, and the season's infectious joy opens us to new experiences and new people. That joy can be heard in the laughter of flirting couples and playing children. Spring's life-affirming shout has relaxed into abundant and easy laughter, the sound of summer.

The heart may be the seat of love, but Eastern medicine also draws a connection between the heart and mind, and so do many of the metaphors we use in everyday speech, such as "my heart wasn't in it" or "in my heart, I didn't believe him." The heart, in Eastern thought, is not just a pump that pushes blood around our body but is part of our inner intelligence, enabling us to be intuitive and insightful. We sense, assess, and judge with our heart. In fact, the Chinese word for heart, *xin*, is often translated as "heart-mind." In Eastern traditions, the heart chakra, our center of intuition and emotion, lies behind the solar plexus. As we speak, we may unconsciously put our hand there to emphasize that we are being sincere and earnest. The heart is considered the arbiter of what is real and false, good and bad.

Summertime is also the perfect season for new babies. The human mating season is in the fall, so each summer naturally brings a surge in the number of newborns. We are still affected by this ancient cycle, which once ensured that our very helpless offspring arrived when temperatures were warm and food was plentiful. If you or someone you know is the mother of a new infant, this is a wonderful time to bond with the child and create a peaceful, joyous environment for it to experience. Make sure an infant is well protected from the fire of the sun, but he or she will be especially fortunate to come into the world during the season of the heart.

The rituals of summer are designed to open, release, and expand your physical and subtle body, encouraging the flow of joy and love that should come naturally to you during this time of year. They are also designed to balance the powerful influence of fire, allowing you to experience its benefits without exhausting your *chi*. This is not important only for your comfort and health during the summer. The effects of such depletion and excess heat will be felt later in the year, when your Body-Mind is unable to cool down with the return of yin in the autumn. It is important to use natural means to cool the body during the summer instead of just relying on air-conditioning. If you are active outdoors, stay in the shade as much as possible. Wear light, loosely woven, natural-fiber clothing that breathes. Moving back and forth from frigid air-conditioned interiors to the torrid heat of outdoors is shocking to the system and can bring about colds and flu.

REMOVING YOUR ARMOR

Summer's glorious sun invites us to shed our clothes, put on a swimsuit, and enjoy its warm rays. As we discussed in our rituals for spring, this often causes us to reevaluate our physical body. Instead of thinking only about weight and shape, I'd like you to think about the way you hold your body—what you're doing with it when you stand and sit and move. Remember, the habits of your physical body affect your subtle body as well. We spend a great deal of time thinking about our bumps and bulges and the fact that our ankles are too thick or our bottom too flat. This is the time to look at what underlies all that and to think about the meaning of your body language.

Our posture speaks volumes about us. You've probably known a woman who "carried" herself exceptionally well, who expressed great body confidence when she entered a room and seemed to be very fluid and at ease when she moved. Her size was unimportant, and she radiated charisma—an expression of power—from her center outward. This marvelous quality can and does flow from a Body-Mind that is unimpeded by chakra blockages. Similarly, the familiar rounded-shoulder, curled-in posture of many women expresses feelings of weakness, uncertainty, smallness, and even neediness. When we stand this way, we are collapsing in around two important energy centers, the first of which governs creativity and communication (the throat chakra) and the second, love and compassion (the heart chakra). Since the heart is the organ that corresponds with summer in Eastern medicine, the ritual that follows will help bring you into balance with the unique energy of this time of year.

Stress can create areas of chronic muscular tension, sometimes referred to as "armoring." The inability to express emotion—whether it's fear, anger, or anxi-

ety—often leads to this condition. The same muscles we use to express an emotion will tighten and contract if we repress that emotion. If we think about where
our "armor" feels heaviest, many of us identify our upper body. In Eastern medicine, this part of our body is associated with responsibility, work, and the perceptions of the outside world. The vast majority of people visiting our spa cite
the upper back, neck, and shoulders as their primary "stress zone," where muscles
are in a near-constant state of tension. A bit more exploration by their massage
therapist usually reveals that this tightness extends to the scalp and facial muscles
as well as to the hips and sacrum.

The neck, face, head, and scalp are the location of the throat, brow, and crown
chakras respectively, so armoring in this area tends to relate to the activities governed by these three energy centers—self-expression and communication, self-
awareness, and even spiritual consciousness. By dropping our armor we can reac-
tivate the flow of energy through these chakras, opening ourselves for physical
and emotional healing.

To perform this ritual effectively, you'll need to stop reading at the end of this
first set of instructions. Read the instructions through three times and absorb
them completely. Continue the ritual and read on after you have opened your
eyes.

- Take a moment and stand in front of a mirror. Stand with your feet shoulder-width apart and close your eyes.
- Drop your shoulders and roll them back slightly to open your chest. Focus
your awareness on any resistance you feel in your body. Envision your heart
chakra warming the muscles of the chest with its glow, loosening and freeing
them.
- Now pretend an invisible filament is pulling you up from the top of your
head, separating your rib cage from your lower abdomen. Envision this filament drawing you up off the ground into the sky, letting your body hang
freely and stretch.

- Inhale deeply, counting to three, feeling air expand your lungs from top to bottom. Wait a second, then exhale slowly, counting to six as you do. Repeat this breathing cycle six times. Then bring you awareness to your body and the change in its energy.
- Hold this posture for about a minute. While you are in this posture, think about how it feels. How do you imagine it would look to a passerby? How do you imagine it would look to someone who knows you well?
- Now open your eyes and carefully observe how you appear in the mirror.

When you opened your eyes, what did you find? Observing the appearance of this strange-feeling posture in the mirror usually reveals not an exaggerated, aggressive-looking stance but simply a woman standing up reasonably straight! In most cases, you'll notice that your body looks remarkably relaxed for all the effort you've gone to. People with curled-in posture cause their muscles to shorten, making it literally feel like a "stretch" to just stand normally. That reinforces the sensation of comfort in the unnatural curled-in position—so the vicious circle goes on.

There are several ways to address poor postural habits more aggressively: bodywork, exercise, and movement therapy. Bodywork can offer near-miraculous results for postural imbalance. This type of muscular tension responds well to a range of intense deep-pressure modalities, including neuro-muscular massage, Shiatsu, myofascial trigger-point therapy, and Rolfing. These aforementioned modalities can be uncomfortable, even painful (Rolfing and myofascial release manipulations can easily bring tears to your eyes), but they have the ability to break through armor and restore the natural symmetry and balance of the body, even cure debilitating headaches. Two forms of movement therapy, the Feldenkrais and Pilates methods, offer excellent results. Feldenkrais is a gentle, remarkably subtle form of body-awareness and movement therapy that restores a healthy neuromuscular response. Pilates training, which began as a type of rehabilitation for injured dancers, emphasizes proper postural alignment and body awareness, emanating from the center of the body, the all-important "girdle" of muscles that support and surround the back and abdomen.

Remember, it took your body a long time to develop its armor. It takes a while to remove it. Getting through the armor takes a variety of modalities, like balneotherapy, meditation, yoga, and self-massage. But simple awareness, too, is key. This ritual of body awareness should be repeated frequently to remind you of any negative postural habits that are contributing to armoring. By regularly removing your armor, you will find that you are standing and moving with greater ease and confidence, and that your heart chakra is fully open to the energies of the season.

BODY CONTOURING MASSAGE

Summer is a natural weight-loss season because it is our period of peak activity. We are designed to carry less weight in the summertime and add weight in the winter. Our bodies are naturally slimmed and toned from the activity of summer.

However, when we confront the prospect of putting on a swimsuit, many of us would like to feel a bit firmer or have our body contours smoother. Our lifestyle is typically more sedentary than that of our ancestors. Even if you work out, if you spend a great deal of your life seated in front of a computer, your lymphatic and blood circulation is affected. Your body can be reshaped by habitual armoring, but it's also reshaped by inadequate circulation. Processed foods, synthetic hormonal additives in meat and dairy products, and foods containing toxic residue from chemical pesticides all contribute greatly to the figure imbalance we call cellulite.

Many women mistakenly think they have cellulite, because another condition common to the upper legs, "deep-tissue dehydration," looks similar to the untrained eye. To tell if the uneven texture you're observing is cellulite, firmly run your fingertips from the inside of the knee upward, stroking across the thigh toward the groin. This follows the lymph channels in the upper legs. You can actually *feel* cellulite, which often forms hard adhesions and nodules under the skin.

Deep-tissue dehydration causes the orange-peel texture on the backs of the thighs. It will usually display a horizontal pattern, and if you lift the skin slightly upward, the uneven texture will disappear. (Not so with cellulite.) The skin sags for two reasons: one, because the muscle underneath has shrunk (atrophied from lack of nourishment), and two, because the skin lacks water in the connective tissues. This is due to a lack of mineral salts, which attract and bind water in the skin. Replacing these vital mineral salts through sea mineral baths (such as the detoxifying balneotherapy ritual described on page 35,) or sea mineral wraps and internal supplements can bring about a quick and gratifying improvement in this condition. Then exercise and massage can tone the underlying muscle.

Fortunately, cellulite responds to a program of detoxification, stimulated both internally and externally, as well as a combination of specialized and precise deep tissue and lymphatic massage to break up adhesions and drain stagnant fluids. Massage therapist Charles W. Wiltsie III, LMT, NCTMB, conducted an unprecedented year-long study proving that specific deep tissue massage, which he calls Lypossage, can help healthy women reduce body dimensions without losing weight. A body-contouring massage helps move toxins out of the targeted areas of the body through lymphatic drainage. Increased circulation nourishes and improves muscle tone. The thighs, buttocks, and lower stomach are particularly apt to respond because they contain a great deal of fatty tissue, lymphatic vessels, and visceral organs that eliminate waste. They also contain some of the largest muscles in the body.

The best result is achieved when self-massage is used as maintenance after you've been treated by a therapist who uses one of these techniques. It's difficult to perform an effective self-massage on the back of the leg or buttocks; it's not possible to achieve all the leverage needed to work the less accessible areas. But you can still benefit from a self-administered program of massage strokes and manipulations.

By increasing the health of the muscles and lymph, you receive a wonderful aesthetic benefit, that of smoothing and contouring. But body-contouring massage also supports nature's detoxifying work and its nurturing effects enhance Body-Mind balance. And in keeping with our summertime instinct to bare our bodies and enjoy the sunshine, this ritual helps us feel better about ourselves when we put on a swimsuit.

There are six basic massage strokes, and each varies in depth depending on the area worked and the result desired. This self-massage ritual itself takes about twenty minutes. For the fastest results, do three treatments a week for six weeks.

Caution: Do not perform this ritual if you have any varicose veins, blood clots, or are pregnant.

- Begin by establishing a positive intention for the treatment. This is not about fixing a "bad" body. Use this affirmation: I love my body and I'm taking good care of it.
- Blend an ounce of jojoba oil with 2 drops each of grapefruit, clary sage, and fennel essential oils. Clary sage is a euphoric with benefits for the reproductive system; cellulite is aggravated by hormonal imbalance. Clary sage stimulates creativity and releases inhibition; however, it should not be used before driving or activities requiring mental focus. Fennel is often used by aromatherapists in the treatment of PMS. Grapefruit is cleansing and detoxifying with mild diuretic properties. Warm the oil in the glass beaker of an electric coffeemaker or use a baby-bottle warmer.
- Take a shower to warm and prepare the skin.

• Dry off.

• *Effleurage: Caution.* Be sure to test the temperature of the oil before dispensing it! This is a long, sweeping stroke of the entire open hand that's used to stimulate circulation and lymphatic drainage. It's also relaxing and calming. Effleurage is performed with a light application of oil. Beginning at the ankles, slide your hands upward, hand over hand, toward the lymph nodes behind your knees. Then move up the thigh, sweeping hand over hand toward the groin area, also the site of lymph nodes. *Always* massage toward the heart. Spend one minute on each leg.

• *Petrissage.* This stroke is shorter than effleurage and is done with fingers, palms, and thumbs. Its strokes are similar to effleurage strokes except they are more narrow and smaller. Because when massaging yourself your hands are essentially backward compared to those of someone else working on your body, you can perform a variation on this technique by making loose fists and using the flat surfaces between your knuckles to perform the strokes. Strokes can be used to focus on target areas. After working each leg for about a minute, you should begin to see some reddening of the skin as circulation is stimulated. At this point, a good deal of the jojoba oil should have absorbed into the skin. If there is excess, wipe it off with a towel. You'll need some "grip" for the next phase.

• *Skin rolling.* This is the lifting of the skin in bunches between fingers and thumbs and then rolling the skin. It is a difficult technique. However, it's effective in breaking up adhesions, softening fascia, improving muscle tone, and stimulating circulation. It is a vigorous technique that requires some skill to prevent discomfort and bruising. Begin very gently. Use both hands to work the front and sides of the thighs and even the soft, loose tissue of the lower belly. Be very careful when working on your abdomen. Lie on your side to massage the buttocks with one hand and roll onto your back to reach the backs of the thighs, again using both hands. The lifting of the skin is important because you're attempting to loosen adhesions. You will build up a tolerance for any discomfort as tissue becomes healthier and more flexible and circulation is enhanced. Even if you have a tendency to form small bruises at first, if you persist with the treatments your skin will become more resilient and these will not continue to occur. Spend three minutes working each side of your lower body.

• *Tapotement.* This is the "chopping" technique you see in the movies when the boxer is on the table getting a massage. The key to this technique is endurance. It needs to be done in the target areas for two to three minutes, which is harder than it sounds. Do not use this technique on your stomach or lower back, where you could injure the kidneys. To treat the back of the legs, sit in a chair and rest your foot against the edge of a desk or tabletop.

• *Deep kneading.* Now we can begin to slow down. The stimulating phase of the treatment is over. Apply a small amount of the warm oil. Deep kneading is a relatively easy stroke that involves gathering skin in the palms of the hands and kneading it like bread dough. It is good for circulation and muscle tone. Spend about two minutes on each leg.

• *Compression.* This is a wonderful technique that can help ease edema. It is simply compressing a target area with open hands for about a minute. Follow with light effleurage toward the lymph nodes on the backs of the legs and the groin, and it will help to drain the lymphatic system. Spend about two minutes on each side of the body.

• When you've finished the massage, take another shower and thoroughly cleanse all the oil from your skin. Soak in a warm, detoxifying seaweed bath (see spring's Detoxifying Seaweed Bath). This will help complete the lymphatic cleansing process.

• Over the next twenty-four hours, drink lots of water to help flush waste out of your system. Dislodged lymphatic waste ends up in the circulatory system, where it is filtered out by the kidneys. Adequate hydration is essential to this process. Drink small amounts of room-temperature or warm fluid frequently rather than taking large glasses of water.

Congratulations! You've completed a sophisticated spa treatment that will yield gratifying results when repeated in a series of twenty, three times per week.

SUMMER TEA-TIME RITUAL

With the summer's increase in fire energy, heat increases in our bodies. However, our digestive fires are not strong at this time of year. When people remark that the heat "kills their appetite," they are sensing weaker digestive energy. Cool foods and beverages seem more appetizing. A hot summer day and an ice-cold drink with your meal: What could be better?

Wait! Those weak digestive fires will be extinguished altogether by that iced tea or ice water. Cooling your body is a question of balancing outer and inner heat. Taking warm showers and even drinking hot liquids will help you sweat, which can cool the body by equalizing the temperature inside and outside. Cold food and beverages can cause sudden contraction and tightening, preventing heat from dispersing from the body or even bringing digestion to an abrupt halt. Water is best consumed at room temperature or warmer, and one of the best sources of water in your diet is fruits and vegetables, preferably those that are organically grown.

Water consumption should increase during the summer. Though most of us have been raised on the standard of "eight 8-ounce glasses of water a day," the best way to drink water is in small amounts, about three or four ounces at a time. This is particularly true with meals, when it's important to keep your digestive enzymes at full strength. In Chinese medicine, excessive water consumption is believed to increase yin energy, making us feel cold and even weak. If you've noticed that you have a hard time staying warm, even in the summer, you may actually be drinking too much water. Common sense is the best guide to determining your ideal water consumption rate. The Zen maxim "Eat when hungry, drink when thirsty" probably says it all.

Peppermint, chamomile, green tea, or raspberry leaf tea, brewed in advance and served hot, warm, or at room temperature, is a surprisingly pleasant accompaniment during fire season. All have astringent properties that make them naturally cooling, and teas supply the hard-to-find astringent taste for your sensory-balanced meal. Raspberry leaf tea helps calm sugar cravings. It can supply energy without creating jitters, so it makes a good substitute for coffee and caffeinated teas. It is also thought to ease hormonal imbalance in women.

This simple tea ritual will help ease excessive heat during fire season. These seasonal flowers create a beautiful tea that is fragrant even when consumed warm, and help to balance you when the body is retaining heat.

Purchase these ingredients from a quality tea or herb purveyor. Imperial Tea Court in San Francisco's Chinatown sells its fine teas by mail. (See Resources.) Freshness is paramount. Store your tea in tightly sealed opaque containers, as they are delicate and easily ruined by both moisture and light.

YOU WILL NEED:
A handful of best quality dry chrysanthemum blossoms
(from a Chinese herbalist)
A handful of best quality dry honeysuckle blossoms
(from a Chinese herbalist)
Jasmine pearl tea (12 pearls)
32 ounces purified or filtered water (not distilled)
A teapot and a steeping pot

• The above recipe is a combination of different teas that steep at different temperatures. When your water boils, put the chrysanthemum and honeysuckle flowers into a pot and allow them to steep for 3 to 4 minutes. You can allow them to steep longer for a more intense tea, but begin with a shorter period. Pour off the water after steeping, into a teapot. (Reserve the flowers; you can reuse them at least once more if you simply store them in the refrigerator. You'll need to use more hot water and longer steeping the second time.) The water must cool a bit before steeping jasmine tea, which due to its delicacy prefers lower temperatures. If you can put your finger in the water without quickly withdrawing it, the temperature is perfect for steeping jasmine. This tea can be enjoyed lukewarm and room temperature as well. Remove the blossoms if you plan to keep any of the brewed tea, but if you are just making a cupful, you can leave them in.

• Select a special cup for your tea. A neutral or white glaze is good when you're getting to know your tea; it helps you gauge its strength.

• Choose a sacred space to enjoy your tea. A thermos lets you turn any garden or park into your own tea garden. Or retreat to a quiet, uncluttered room with a comfortable chair and a window to open for fresh air.

TEATIME CONTEMPLATION ON THE SENSES

• Smell: Enjoy the fragrance; the exotic perfume of this tea cools the overheated, overactive mind and encourages quiet contemplation.

• Taste: Savor the delicacy and complexity of this blend, which rivals that of a fine wine. Taste it as you would wine, holding it in your mouth gently and letting it roll over the sides of the tongue. The nuances of flavor are captivating.

• Sight: The leaves of these tea plant tips are hand rolled into tiny pearls, which magically unfurl after several minutes of steeping.

• Touch: The mild warmth of the teacup in the hand is a comforting, calming sensation.

• Sound: The sound of tea is silence: It is the beverage of contemplation and reverie.

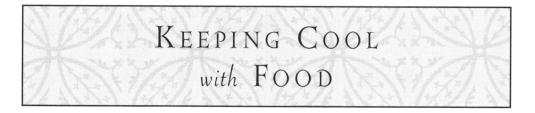

KEEPING COOL *with* FOOD

The "warming," tissue-building foods of winter, like meat, eggs, nuts, and cheese should be eaten in moderation during the summertime. Your diet now should be rich with the bountiful fruits and vegetables of the season.

Bitter flavors have a cooling effect, which can be very beneficial during the summer. In Chinese medicine, excess heat is thought to become trapped in the body, only to return later in the year as fever. Infection and inflammation can be positively affected by introducing the bitter flavor to the Body-Mind. The heart, the organ associated with summer, is thought to be cleared of heat by bitter tastes. No wonder we may crave a big salad of bitter greens for dinner when the weather is hot and sultry!

Cooling Summer Chopped Salad

This light summer salad can be a dinner or an accompaniment. If possible, choose greens that have grown in your region; they're more seasonally attuning. The fresher, the better—and, of course, nothing beats lettuces picked from your garden. While the bitter flavor is showcased in this salad, it is gently balanced by the sweet, represented by the lemon cucumber, pepper, eggs, and honey. In this recipe, you chop the radicchio and include lime zest in the dressing to help distribute the bitter flavor evenly through the salad. If you can, prepare the dressing about an hour in advance to let the basil infuse into the olive oil.

Juice and zest of two limes
1 tablespoon honey
A loose handful of fresh basil leaves,
finely chopped
2 tablespoons extra virgin olive oil
1 head of romaine lettuce, chopped
1 cup of radicchio leaves, coarsely chopped
2 green onions, chopped
1 sweet red bell pepper, chopped
1 lemon cucumber, coarsely chopped
2 hard-boiled eggs, chopped
Salt and pepper to taste

1. Whisk together the lime juice and zest, honey, and basil. Drizzle in olive oil and whisk until ingredients are emulsified. Set aside, preferably keeping the dressing at room temperature to ensure flavors are at their peak and encourage the infusion of the basil's natural oils.

2. Wash and dry the lettuces. Mix together the romaine, radicchio, green onions, bell pepper, cucumber, and egg.

3. Add the dressing and toss thoroughly. Serve with a warm, crusty whole grain roll and sweet butter.

Heat Balancing Salsa

Surprisingly, spicy foods are also recommended during hot weather. They help to balance external and internal heat. This moderately spicy salsa uses the fresh fruit of the season as well as garlic, ginger, onion, and jalapeño pepper, which helps to equalize internal and external heat. Mix ingredients quickly together. Spoon this salsa over broiled fish or steamed summer vegetables. Or enjoy it with flavorful stone-ground corn tortilla chips, like Barbara's Pinta Chips, available at your natural foods store.

1 lemon, peeled and sectioned

1 grapefruit, peeled and sectioned

2 limes, peeled and sectioned

1 avocado, diced

1 mango, diced

2 tablespoons raspberry conserves

2 cloves garlic, chopped

2 tablespoons minced pickled ginger (Japanese condiment)

1 red onion, chopped

1 jalapeño pepper, minced

This salsa should be used immediately as it does not store well.

Breakfast for a Hot Summer Day

This is one of the best breakfasts for ensuring that you won't become irritable and peevish when summer's fire causes your internal heat to rise. Nutty flavored, chewy brown rice has a delicious sweet flavor and excellent detoxifying properties. It is full of B vitamins, which makes it a wonderful food for the nervous system, particularly if you're undergoing stress. Your rice can be baking while you complete your wake-up rituals, pages 108–114.

In Ayurveda, it's believed that milk has great nourishing and strengthening properties. It's known for its ability to cool fire energy and to calm nerves caused by excess air energy. Ayurvedic practitioners recommend boiling even pasteurized milk to ensure that it is easy to digest. Whole milk is one of Ayurveda's important healing foods and is considered healthier for you than our popular reduced-fat and nonfat milk. If you plan to drink milk, make sure you use organic products.

1/3 cup organic whole milk, boiled

1/2 cup organic brown rice

1/2 teaspoon organic ghee (found in your
natural foods market)

1 1/4 cups boiling water

1/8 teaspoon sea salt

Pinch of cinnamon

Pinch of ginger

4 dried apricots, chopped

Boil milk briefly and set aside. Sauté rice in ghee until it begins to brown. This will intensify the nutty flavor. Transfer to a small baking dish and pour boiling water over it. Cover the dish and bake for 40 to 45 minutes, or until all the water is absorbed. Sprinkle spices and chopped apricots over the top. Pour milk over it. Serves one.

A Simple Red Feast for Summer

The color of the season, red, evokes passion and love. Use this vibrant recipe whenever you'd like to feel more energetic, happy, or affectionate. It is full of the red hue and a simple way to help attune yourself to the energy of summer. It's also a perfect one-dish summer meal when you're in the mood for something light.

1 pound fresh salmon fillet (serves two)

2 sweet peppers

1 pound vine-ripe tomatoes

1/2 pound arugula

1/2 pound spinach leaves, well washed and patted dry

FOR THE DRESSING:

2 tablespoons fresh lime juice

2 tablespoons rice vinegar

3 tablespoons organic clover honey

1 teaspoon chopped fresh mint

Finely minced zest of one lemon

2 tablespoons very finely minced red bell pepper

¹/₃ cup plain organic yogurt

¹/₄ cup hazelnut oil

1. Broil or poach the salmon fillet up to a day in advance, remove skin, and chill thoroughly.

2. Choose vivid red and orange sweet peppers, and vine-ripe tomatoes in the same hues. You may want to steam the peppers lightly to make them easier to digest, then let them cool to room temperature.

3. Create a bed of fresh arugula and spinach on a serving platter. Place the salmon on top of the greens and add the peppers and tomatoes. The cooling bitterness of the greens will complement the sweetness of the salmon, peppers, and tomatoes.

4. This sweet dressing is good for balancing heat. Sour flavors can aggravate fire, so vinegar and citrus should be sweetened slightly. The most important thing is that the flavor of the dressing be *predominantly* sweet, not sour.

5. Whisk together the lime juice, rice vinegar, honey, mint, lemon zest, red bell pepper, and yogurt. Whisk in the hazelnut oil last, ensuring that the mixture is smooth. The red bell pepper imparts an unusual delicate pink color to the dressing.

6. Pour dressing over the salmon and the greens.

7. For dessert, serve a lavish array of perfectly ripe cherries, apricots, nectarines, watermelon, cantaloupe, and papaya. These fruits protect against and treat excessive heat. No wonder watermelon is so refreshing in the summer!

An Altar *to* Joy

The sacred space of the summer is the shared space where we come together with friends and loved ones. To create a very special ritual of joy, you can transform your dinner or lunch table into an altar that celebrates the senses and delights the imagination. Ayurvedic philosophy holds that simply gazing at something beautiful will calm summer's excessive fire energy. By creating a beautiful setting for summertime meals, you will create balance for yourself and your guests.

Allow plenty of time to gather the materials for your altar. The fun and discovery of creating a beautiful setting is just as important as the meal you enjoy there. If it becomes a chore, it will lose its magic and its benefit to you. Sharing the preparation process makes this ritual even more seasonally attuning: Summer is the ideal time for group activities. Enjoy the synergy of creating something special with others.

- If you can, create your altar in a garden, on a terrace, or on a lawn. Placing a table in an unexpected spot refreshes the eye and rearranges expectations. A beautifully set table outdoors makes a meal that much more of a treat.
- Drape your table with a generous swath of lovely fabric. If it's hot and sultry, light and pastel colors are the most cooling to the eye. A layer of sheer fabric can also give a magical sense of lightness.
- Create an oversized, low flower arrangement for your table using a variety of red, pink, and orange-hued flowers arranged in a wreath. Among the flowers, weave jasmine vine, ivy, and blackberries or tiny wine grapes still on their stems. In the center, nestle a basket mounded with still more fabulously ripe summer fruit, interspersed with single blossoms. Around the centerpiece cluster an array of softly colored votive-style candles in a variety of heights.

• Tie crisp, oversized white linen napkins with long sprigs of creeping rosemary and tuck a flower into each. Use your best flatware, but mix it with a cheerful jumble of glassware and colorful mismatched plates—or paper plates.

• When you sit down at your table to eat, take several deep breaths and allow yourself to absorb the visual beauty of the altar as well as the animated faces of your companions as they respond to it.

• Music is the language of summer, so to add a special audio element to your altar, hide a portable stereo somewhere in the foliage. Better yet, invite musically inclined friends to share your meals. A personal performance is the ultimate summertime experience—and the perfect homage to the season.

SUMMER MORNING MEDITATION

While we don't want to encourage a full-fledged return to sun worship, it's unfortunate that these days the sun is regarded almost purely as a threat to our well-being. Sunlight, the same light that gives us life, is also the harbinger of ultraviolet damage and free radicals that can cause freckles, wrinkles, and more serious skin damage. Nevertheless, there are many ways to enjoy the summer sun in moderation.

We get vitamin D from sunlight, and most of us who work indoors don't receive enough. Both vitamin D and magnesium are essential for calcium absorption, a nutritional benefit especially valuable to women. Nutritional expert Paul Pitchford tells us in his book *Healing with Whole Foods* that exposing twenty percent of the body to the sun for thirty minutes at sea level provides us with the vitamin D we need for proper calcium absorption. (Our faces and hands comprise only about five percent of the body's surface area.)

Keep in mind, however, that sun protection is essential. Here are some guidelines that will allow you to enjoy the sun while protecting fragile skin:

- Sunscreen must be fresh—the active ingredients in that bottle of sunscreen left over from last year have expired.
- Sunscreen must be applied copiously, not sparingly. It must be reapplied frequently, especially if you're perspiring or in the water.
- Always apply sun protection at least a half hour before exposure. The ingredients don't become fully active until they've been absorbed by the skin.
- If you also have sun allergies and get rashes from sun exposure, a sign of excess fire energy, use a sunblock that contains titanium dioxide or zinc oxide.

A small amount of early morning sun can be beneficial for most of us. If you enjoy morning walks or like to go for a run when the sun is just rising, you've probably enjoyed the limpid quality of light that's unique to the early morning. It expands and opens your heart with the fresh promise of the new day. Summer's excess fire energy is beautifully balanced by morning sun. For someone who loves to sleep, the early morning sun helps to counteract sluggishness and infuses the Body-Mind with the lively energy of the season.

In most Eastern traditions, it's considered important to get up in time to enjoy the sunrise. Observing the sunrise or early morning sun offers us a quiet moment to collect our thoughts for the day. Getting up in a rush and hurrying off exacerbates our fire energy and can contribute to a feeling of being overwhelmed. This is a lovely, easy ritual that you can perform to soak up the sun's therapeutic rays without risking sunburn and more insidious skin damage:

- Bathe, do your basic morning ablutions, and throw on some comfortable clothes. Choose light or bright colors. If you're a dyed-in-the-wool urban black-wearer, try replacing black, which is the absence of all color, with white—which includes every wavelength of light in the spectrum. This can literally brighten your outlook on the new day.

• Place a comfortable straight-backed chair outside, if possible, or next to a window. You can also sit on the ground or the floor, cross-legged. If you sit on the floor, put a folded towel under your tailbone to help open the lower abdomen and allow the legs to be below the hips. Ideally, you should face the sun.

• Put a drop or two of undiluted lemon and geranium aromatic oils on a pure cotton handkerchief; these essences will help to awake and enliven you. Fruit oils like lemon have *high, light* notes that facilitate the flow of mental energy and are also known as *head notes*. Geranium oil, like the season of summer, has the most balanced blend of yin and yang energy. Interestingly, it is neither stimulating nor relaxing. Hold the scented handkerchief to your face and take several deep breaths through your nose. Then set it aside for the breathing exercise.

• Pranayama, or alternate nostril breathing, is a yoga practice designed for your morning ritual. Close your eyes, putting your right hand up to your face, thumb beside your right nostril, and two middle fingers beside your left nostril. Don't extend your elbow outward; let it rest against your side, unsupported by your chair. This practice begins on the exhalation.

Press your right nostril gently shut with your thumb, exhaling through your left nostril. Inhale just a little more deeply and slowly than normal, keeping the right nostril closed.

Now gently press shut your left nostril, using your two middle fingers; exhale just a bit more slowly than normal.

• Alternate breathing through each nostril for about 4 to 5 minutes. After you complete this cycle, pick up the handkerchief and conclude by taking a few easy breaths of the aromatic essences. Feel the sensation of awakening flowing through your entire body. Now that your lungs have expanded and your circulatory system has been awakened, move into the following classic series of yoga postures, specifically designed to help you begin your day in balance. This routine is beneficial year-round.

SALUTATION *to the* SUN

If you've explored yoga before, you've probably encountered the Salutation to the Sun, a series of postures that are practiced in the morning. It is a curiously habit-forming holistic exercise that provides stimulation and integration for the entire Body-Mind. Besides increasing circulation to the muscles, the postures lubricate the joints and vertebrae. It is also said to "massage" the internal organs.

The Salutation to the Sun is performed in cycles, and the goal is to achieve fluidity and ease as you transition gracefully from one posture to the next. There are twelve different postures in all. At first, it may be hard to think about your breathing while you're concentrating on the postures. After practice, the pattern of inhalation and exhalation becomes quite natural.

If you've been sedentary, these postures, though simple in appearance, can be challenging. Of course, if you watch an experienced yoga practitioner performing Salutation to the Sun, it looks nearly effortless, almost like the rippling of water. Keeping this image of ease and fluidity in mind, begin very slowly. Never strain or push yourself. Make sure that you breathe regularly, as holding your breath will cause strain and possibly injury. A complete exhalation allows your muscles to relax and extends your range of motion.

Breath, the source of life, is the key to experiencing the benefits of yoga. Along with the food that we eat, the air that we breathe creates us. In Ayurveda, the breath is the means by which *prana*, or the life force, enters our body. Breath animates both our physical and our subtle body; our breathing responds to our emotional state, becoming shallow and uneven when we're stressed. However, it also works in reverse: by taking deep, even breaths we can reduce anxiety and clear our minds.

Most of us do not know how to expand our lungs when we breathe and tend to inhale into just the upper portion of the lung. Similarly, we seldom exhale fully and allow the lungs to be completely cleansed. Yogic breathing helps us become aware of the upper, middle, and lower lung. The diaphragm/solar plexus area corresponds with the third chakra, which is associated with the nervous system and governs our raw emotional energy. Breathing exercises that fill and empty the lower lung offer us the opportunity to balance and optimize both the physical and the subtle body.

In yoga, exhalations accompany stretching, opening, and elongating movements. This is an easy way to remember what to do with your breath as you practice the poses. By contrast, inhalations—contracting from the belly—accompany bending, folding, and closing.

First posture: Stand tall, imagining a filament pulling you from the top of your head upward. Your feet should be parallel and close together, though not touching. Put your hands together, palm to palm, fingers pointing upward in a "prayer" position close to your chest. Looking straight ahead, slowly begin to inhale, lifting your rib cage.

Second posture: As you inhale, lift your arms directly up, rotating your palms outward and upward as you near complete extension. Let your eyes follow your hands upward, but don't focus on them. At the top, your palms will be facing the ceiling, thumbs turned inward. Your hands will end up slightly behind your head so that your spine is flexing very gently backward as you look up.

Third posture: Begin your exhalation, bending forward with arms still extended (you can relax and bend your knees; don't lock them) and bring your hands to the floor. Keep your upper body and arms loose. You will feel a stretch in your calves; don't force it. As your hands touch the floor, allow your palms to make full contact as you . . .

Fourth posture: . . . inhale and extend your left leg behind you, like a runner in a starting block. Plant your hands firmly, fingers pointed outward for support. This movement may feel a little awkward to you at first. Let the knee of the extended leg touch the ground. Your right leg will be bent, the foot flat. This leg must be perpendicular to your foot. You may need to make an adjustment to straighten it. Imagine your spine extending outward in both directions, lifting your chin without bending back at the neck. Your chest should be filled with breath as you let your gaze follow through along the line created by your spine.

Fifth posture: Exhale, bringing the front leg back beside the left leg. From this push-up–like position you immediately begin to raise your hips, pressing into the floor with the palms of your hands, which you now place securely hip-width apart, fingers forward, flat. Your feet should be no farther apart than your hips. As you exhale, pressing into the floor with your hands and feet, imagine being lifted upward from your hips by a crane. Keep your head and neck relaxed. You will feel a strong hamstring stretch.

Sixth posture: Continuing your exhalation, release from the strong upward extension and let your elbows bend and hands slide forward to allow your forearms to touch the floor. Let your knees drop softly down, feet sliding back slightly, and continue smoothly rolling downward until toes, knees, thighs, forearms, and forehead all make contact with the floor for a brief moment as you flow into . . .

Seventh posture: . . . the Cobra pose. Inhale as you gently push up your chest and shoulders, pressing into the floor with your hands, arms tucked close to your sides, and tightening your buttocks to protect your lower back from strain. This posture's upward extension should originate in your pelvis, not your upper body. Extend your neck and head upward and outward, letting your shoulders fall away.

Eighth posture: Now the cycle begins in reverse, with an exhalation. Raise your hips upward, pushing into the floor with the hands, back into the fifth posture. Try to push the heels down into the floor. Your head should be relaxed.

Ninth posture: With an inhalation, return to the fourth posture. This requires bringing the right foot forward and placing it between your hands. For beginners this is sometimes accomplished with a little "hop," lowering your body back into the "runner's" position. Your left leg is now extended behind you, its knee lightly contacting the floor for balance. Your left leg should be perpendicular to the floor; adjust it if necessary. Remember to extend and elongate the spine, lifting your chest as you inhale.

Tenth posture: Now you can bring your left leg forward to place your feet side by side, remaining loosely bent over with your arms extended downward. Keep your hands on the floor; if you need to relax your knees to touch the floor, that's fine. In this posture you are exhaling. Your head and arms are aligned with the spine.

Eleventh posture: Roll up, vertebra by vertebra, lifting the body as you inhale, and don't lead with the head. After you return to the standing position, slowly raise your hands over your head and return to the second posture, palms and head facing upward, spine gently flexed backward.

Twelfth posture: As you return to the first posture, the Salutation, lower your arms and exhale. You'll finish with your palms together in front of your chest, elbows loose, spine straight, and eyes facing forward.

After you've concluded the cycle of postures, remain in the first posture, inhaling and exhaling as long as you need to catch your breath. This seemingly gentle series of postures is actually quite rigorous. The first posture now becomes your starting point for the next cycle. Inhale and begin another set. Complete one to six sets, alternating the foot that extends backward as you reach the fourth posture.

When you're finished, lie down and enjoy the sensation of vitality that comes from this marvelous and ancient practice. Every muscle, joint, and nerve seems to be buzzing with energy and awareness. It's a wonderful feeling to start the day with.

SUMMER SWIMMING RITUAL

If time permits, begin with the preceding meditation and yoga practices before moving into a more intensive physical workout. Beginning this way will help with coordination, balance, and focus. You'll find that you breathe easier as you exert yourself, having expanded your lungs fully already with your yoga breathing routine. Your muscles and even your internal organs will be warmed up by the Salutation to the Sun.

Because the fire element is intensified by exercise and exertion, it's important to choose a summertime workout that will enhance your overall state of Body-Mind balance, not just cardiovascular condition or muscle tone. If at all possible, exercise outdoors in the cool morning air. Exercising indoors in an air-conditioned building will not have the same benefit for the Body-Mind, though it is better for you than exercising in the midday sun on a hot summer afternoon. During the summer, we are designed to complete our physical activities earlier in the day, in order to rest during the heat of the day.

One of the best summertime workouts is swimming. Swimming allows you to stay cool and comfortable while enjoying a total Body-Mind workout. It helps to create endurance, muscle strength, and flexibility. And it does all of this while freeing the mind. If you're able to swim in a clean, natural body of water, you'll benefit even more from swimming's restorative properties. Because of its ability to stimulate virtually every sense, swimming is a "total immersion" sensory therapy experience.

• Getting ready: Very important to a successful swimming workout is a comfortable swimsuit. Visit a sporting goods store to choose one that's made for swimming, not sunbathing. If you're swimming in a pool, don't forget your "glamour" accessories: properly fitted goggles and cap. Chlorine is the one drawback of the swimmer's workout. If you're going to be outdoors, make sure you apply a waterproof sunscreen at least thirty minutes before exposure.

• Before you get in the water, take a moment to quietly sit and contemplate it. If you're lucky enough to be the first swimmer of the day, enjoy the sight of the smooth, tranquil surface. The azure color of most pools is very cooling to the Body-Mind; remember, blue is a color that helps put our mind into a meditative state.

• Time your workout instead of counting laps. One of the reasons swimming is so beneficial to you is that it effects a release of the mind! Thirty to forty-five minutes in the pool is excellent. If you're not used to swimming for that long, vary your stroke and slow yourself to ensure that you can stay in motion.

• When you begin, try to swim as slowly as you possibly can, to enable you to focus on the movement of your body. Swimming is an activity that poetically blends yin and yang energy. The active, propelling phase of the stroke expresses your yang energy: dynamic, forward movement, intention, and strength. The floating and gliding phase of the stroke expresses your yin energy, in qualities of passivity, serenity, receptivity, and effortlessness.

• Swimming stimulates the sense of touch more than any other physical activity. The temperature and sensation of the water fully engages the nervous system. To help bring balanced awareness back to your body, concentrate your attention first on your feet, moving upward to the legs, the hips, the lower back, midback, shoulders, arms, hands, head, and neck. At each stage, note what you're feeling. Is there an area of tightness and resistance? If you don't consider yourself a natural swimmer, you may be tense in certain spots, such as your neck, as you try to keep your head above the water to breathe. With each exhalation, breathe tension out through these areas.

• Focus on your breathing and concentrate on bringing air deeply into the lungs, filling the entire lung from bottom to top. Focus on your belly; is it expanding as you inhale? Are you releasing your breath fully, expelling muscular tension?

• Turn your awareness to your range of motion. Extend and stretch your arms and legs while swimming, envisioning smooth and beautiful arcs passing through the water.

• Whenever possible, when you've finished swimming, do this simple ritual to strengthen your legs and begin to "ground" yourself for your return to earth. Walk as fast as you can back and forth across the shallow end of the pool. Repeat about six times. Now stand in the water holding the side of the pool. Contract your abdominal muscles. Lift your right leg out to the side as high as it will comfortably go. Repeat a dozen times, exhaling with a sharp "shhh!" through the exertion, then inhaling through your nose as you bring the leg back down (to milder resistance). Next, lift your right leg slightly to the side and then back in front of your left leg, like a pendulum. Exhale with a "shhh!" as you cross the leg, inhale deeply through the nose as you move your leg back outward. Repeat a dozen times, being careful not to strain. Now repeat with your left leg. By the time you've completed these exercises, which firm and tone the upper legs, you'll be reacquainted with your sense of balance and ready for life back on terra firma.

• Intersperse pool workouts with early morning walks. Walking is a simple, enjoyable, and affordable exercise, and it brings you into contact with the natural world.

AFTER-SWIM SUMMER SKIN CARE

If you swim in a chlorinated pool, you'll need to make sure you cleanse your skin and body thoroughly afterward. Chlorine dries your skin because of its alkalinity; your skin's natural pH is acidic. To remove absorbed chlorine and remoisturize the skin, follow this soothing after-swim ritual:

• The best way to remove chlorine from the skin is to soak in a seaweed algae bath (see spring's Detoxifying Seaweed Bath) The seaweed algae, which has an affinity for chemicals like chlorine, will draw it out of the pores and from the surface layers of the skin. If you don't have time for a soak, take a shower and use a mild, nondetergent aromatherapy body cleanser (see Resources), leaving the cleanser on the skin for a few minutes prior to rinsing, where it will encourage a purge of the follicles and sweat glands. This will help remove chlorine, though a soak is considerably more effective.

• Put a refreshing nonalcoholic toner in a spray bottle and apply it generously over your entire body after showering. Even water's neutral pH is too alkaline for your skin. Not only will toner restore the correct pH to your skin, it will have a delightful cooling effect. While your skin is still damp, you can massage in a superhydrating seaweed algae extract (see Resources), which helps replenish the mineral salts that attract and bind water to the skin. This combination works to eliminate dehydration.

• You still have to emoliate though—remember, hydration and emoliation are two different functions! Seal in moisture with a luxurious nourishing body moisturizer that contains soothing ingredients like wheat germ oil, rich in vitamin E, or shea butter, which contains anti-inflammatory allantoin (see Resources). Another excellent ingredient for a body lotion is lavender essential oil, which is effective for easing minor irritation. Massage the lotion over your entire body using gentle effleurage strokes (see the Body Contouring massage) always working toward the heart. You may want to use a separate, richer product that's designed expressly for the feet, such as a cream that helps exfoliate calluses (see Resources). Be sure to apply plenty of sunscreen if you'll be exposed further that day.

• Do a nasal wash, using a mild saline solution, to soothe the mucous membranes that have been exposed to chlorine. A specially designed Ayurvedic nasal cleansing pitcher, called a Neti pot (see Resources) is an essential self-care tool that makes this very easy. This Neti pot will also come in very handy if you travel to very dry climates, such as high mountains or desert. Follow the instructions on the pot precisely. It can and should be used daily.

• Using a natural eye rinse from the natural foods store after swimming is also helpful. It's difficult to avoid getting any pool water in your eyes even if you use goggles.

WALKING BAREFOOT

Summer activities tend to favor the body while the mind gets easily out of shape. Unfortunately, as we grow older, few of us get to spend our summers at play. Mothers find themselves working harder than ever with school-age children at home during the day. When we're not able to follow our natural instinct to play during the summer, our energy often takes a less constructive path. We may overwork or indulge in pointless worry and obsessive thought patterns. In our summertime thirst for "action," we may find ourselves attracted to strongly stimulating visual imagery, such as summer's blockbuster movies. When yang's aggressive energy is at its peak, exciting or violent imagery becomes more alluring to us. This type of summertime overstimulation can often cause racing thoughts and restlessness.

The sense of touch can be very effective in soothing and slowing the activity of a racing, excitable mind. This is because the skin and the nervous system are deeply intertwined. The tissues of the skin, nervous system, and brain are closely related, having all emerged from the ectoderm during our earliest stages of development. Because of this profound and ancient relationship, the sense of touch creates a powerful link between Mind and Body. When therapeutically applied, it is able to create healthy balance between the two. This ritual uses the sense of touch to ease an overheated mind during the summertime. By treating the feet, we are physically refocusing our energy down and out of our head.

- If you're lucky enough to live near a beach, you should take advantage of the opportunity to walk on the sand barefoot. The sensory stimulation of walking on moist, gritty sand is particularly beneficial for fretfulness and racing thoughts. Walking barefoot on grass will have a similar effect. As the lower terminus for the nervous system, the feet are extraordinarily sensitive and possess reflex points for the entire body. This exercise offers a mild general stimulation of the entire sole of the foot, as opposed to a precise deep pressure on a specific reflex point.

- This is an anti–power walk, a quiet stroll. Focus your awareness on the sensory experience. Stay at a relaxed pace and walk for at least fifteen minutes.

- If you've been experiencing a lot of anxiety or aggression, you'll probably find your pace accelerating as your mind starts to race. Slow down. Don't let your thoughts wander too far from the physical experience. As thoughts pop into your head, gently release them by saying to yourself "that's not important right now." Don't chastise yourself for having a hard time shaking them. Just refocus on the sensation in your feet. Remind yourself quietly that right now, your attention is in your feet, not your head.

• When you return from your walk, complete your ritual by soaking your feet in a tepid (not cold) foot bath containing three drops of lavender essential oil and two drops of tea tree oil. Tea tree, from Australia, has wonderful antifungal properties and is a terrific foot-care ingredient. Soak for about ten minutes, then dry your feet by rubbing them vigorously with a coarse towel.

A SUMMER SANCTUARY
for the HEART

Summer is the season of the heart, but the stress and fatigue of everyday life may rob us of our romantic spirit. This aromatherapy ritual will help open the heart and inspire intimacy in your relationship. This ritual can also be used if you're not in an intimate relationship but would like to be. By opening your heart on this subtle level, you create the optimum conditions for welcoming love into your life. Essential oil of ylang-ylang helps ease feelings of anger and fear and in particular resonates with the heart chakra. Sandalwood is a sensual perfume with a spicy and exotic energy that helps restore our connection with the physical. It helps us break out of old patterns and habits and releases mental inhibitions. Sandalwood's cool, earthy quality grounds us, freeing us from worry and guilt. Neroli is derived from orange blossoms, long a symbol of fertility and feminine allure. It helps evoke a feeling of contentment, relaxation, and safety, facilitating intimacy and easing anxiety.

• Launder bed linens and make up your bed. Remember, this is the sacred space for your loving relationship. Summertime bed linens should be light or bright in color. Pink, pinkish-peach, or rose-colored linens will help you revive romantic energy. The red hue reconnects us to our physical side.

• Apply essential oils directly to pure cotton handkerchiefs and slip them into your freshly laundered pillowcases. Use this blend:

> *3 drops essential oil of ylang-ylang*
> *3 drops essential oil of sandalwood*
> *5 drops essential oil of neroli*

• A bouquet of fresh, beautiful flowers on a bedside table is one of the best ways to keep the spirit of romance alive. If they're from your own garden, so much the better! Roses, sweet peas, freesias, and jasmine, which all have a cooling sweet scent, are wonderful. Exuberant dahlias and peonies, with their sunburst shape and marvelous colors, are seasonally attuning additions to this summer bouquet. Locally grown flowers will be more seasonally attuning, since they are the product of the same environment as you are.

• Don't stage this as a seduction scene. Be open and receptive to any outcome. This is a ritual for creating emotional sanctuary and a deeper sense of intimacy—it has no deadline!

SUMMER LANDSCAPE INFUSION

In *The Yellow Emperor's Classic*, the great sourcebook of Chinese medicine, there are many practices recommended to assure that we remain in harmony with the unique energies of the seasons. Some of them, like the ritual that follows, are deceptively simple.

During summer, our life energy flows outward, expanding and opening. Even the urge to be outdoors is a direct result of this energetic influence. The days are longer; we rise early with the sun and stay up later—though few of us go to sleep when the sun sets, as recommended in Chinese medicine.

Geographically, places that express yang energy are promontories that allow for an expansive view of the landscape. The natural world is at its peak of abundance and growth. The limitless sense that you can "see forever" attunes us with the principle of yang. This is the opposite of the energetic influence of winter, which turns us inward and gathers life into an intimate, smaller circle. Many of us live and work in small spaces. When we are under the influence of summer's fire element, small spaces feel particularly uncomfortable and unnatural. Suddenly, our energy has outgrown our cubicle or apartment. The same is true in urban areas. The energy of the populace swells, and to find relief, city dwellers migrate en masse to the ocean or mountains.

Here is a simple but effective ritual for embracing your expanding yang energy and creating Body-Mind balance during the summer:

• Take a hike to a promontory where you can view the landscape. See if you can find a spot where your view is unobstructed and far-reaching. If you're in an area where you can walk along a ridge, for example, and continuously enjoy the view, all the better. If your vantage point is more restricted, stop there and spend some time taking in the scenery. Even in the city, a tall building with an observation deck can afford some of this same energy. However, simply looking out a window provides too restricted a view, and it's important that you be outdoors.

• As you take in the view, breathe air into your lungs and feel the physical sensation of expansion. Open your chest and lift your rib cage, letting your shoulders drop back and allowing your arms to hang loosely by your sides.

• Try not to focus on any one thing, but keep your field of vision as wide open as possible. If you find yourself adding meaning to anything you see, interpreting, or analyzing, gently stop yourself with the phrase "it's all one," and restore your all-encompassing perspective.

• Because your sense of vision is heightened by fire energy, which in turn excites creativity, you may have the urge to physically respond to the view. A terrific way to do this is to sketch or paint. This can help you deepen your visual experience; however, avoid getting caught up in capturing detail, which shrinks your perspective. For this reason, photography may not be as attuning as expressive media. Recording is not the same as *responding*. Use media that allow you to make sweeping gestures, like charcoal or paint.

HEAT WAVE TEA BATH

Even if you love hot weather, it may not love you back! This remedy is designed to correct the imbalance caused by excessive heat. In Chinese medicine, excess heat absorbed in the summertime is thought to be stored in the body, only to reemerge in wintertime as fever. This gentle bath cure is designed to restore equilibrium, calm, and energy. It's recommended only for very hot weather or when visiting a hot climate.

The best time to do this spa ritual is when you'll have plenty of time to relax afterward, or when you're preparing for bed. You can find teas and herbs in bulk in many natural foods stores. This is the most economical way to purchase them. The green tea has an astringent effect, to help cool and calm inflammation. It's rich in antioxidants, important if you've been overexposed to the sun, the most potent source of free radicals. Oat powder is an excellent antiinflammatory and a superb sunburn treatment. Peppermint cools and soothes, as does lavender essential oil, a mood-lightening aroma. Lavender has the added benefit of being healing and antiseptic as well.

YOU WILL NEED:

2 handfuls loose peppermint tea or dried peppermint leaves
2 handfuls chamomile tea
2 handfuls loose green tea
1 15-inch-diameter piece of cheesecloth cut in a circle
A twist-tie for a large bag
A handful of oat powder, found in your natural foods store
6 drops of lavender essential oil
1 soft, fluffy bath towel
Aloe vera gel
6 drops neroli essential oil

• Lay out the piece of cheesecloth and pour your loose teas in a pile in the center. Bring the edges of the cloth together and create a pouch, twisting the cheesecloth and securing it with the twist-tie. Make sure you don't make the bag too tight; you want the water to circulate through the tea leaves freely—you are creating, in effect, a giant tea bag.

• Draw a hot bath, and as your tub is filling, drop in your tea bag, oat powder, and algae powder. Measure out precisely six drops of lavender essential oil and inhale as the steam lifts this beautiful natural essence toward you. Let your tea "brew" as the bath cools off. You can gently swirl the teabag around a bit to make sure the water circulates through it thoroughly.

• Wait until the water is just a little above skin temperature and then slip into your bath and feel the heat in your body disperse into the mild warmth of the water. (Cool water is too sharp a contrast and will cause contraction, preventing heat from dissipating.) You can allow the water to cool off a bit more as you relax, but don't let yourself become chilled.

• When you get out of the tub, pat your skin dry with a very soft towel. Blend a couple of tablespoons of fresh, high-quality cold-pressed aloe vera gel with neroli oil, and after letting it warm slightly in your hand, massage it gently into your skin. Orange blossom has a soothing effect on the skin and is considered very calming for the Body-Mind. Aloe vera's healing properties are nothing short of remarkable. It is the best sunburn and sun-exposure remedy available. Not only does it soothe and calm, it accelerates your skin's natural healing response dramatically.

• Put on very soft cotton pajamas or loungewear and relax. You should be feeling much more comfortable, but not cold. Be careful not to let yourself get chilled. Avoid iced beverages after the bath; instead, have a cup of peppermint tea.

THE LAUGHING RITUAL

Laughter is the sound stimulated by the fire element, which governs the heart and the season of summer. We associate it with joy, excitement, and happiness; laughter is the natural music of positive and loving energy. A healthy, deep sensation of joy gives rise to a feeling of contentment and delight. Healthy laughter leaves us energized yet relaxed, and when shared, it helps us become more deeply connected to others. Sharing "true" or heartfelt laughter is often part of falling in love or creating profound, lasting friendships. Fire, which governs communication, is the energetic medium of all human relationships, romantic or otherwise, and laughter is its voice.

During summer, laughter is seasonally attuning, helping us achieve the physiological and emotional state we're designed to experience during the season of joy. Laughter increases respiratory activity and also stimulates the production of endorphins, which create a feeling of euphoria and increase our tolerance for pain. No wonder laughter is an instant stress reducer: It floods our bodies with a natural burst of healing chemicals. Given the debilitating effects of stress, this "best medicine" should be taken as often as possible. The following rituals are contraindicated only for people who are prone to excessive amounts of nervous or inappropriate laughter.

Once a week, during the summer, take part in an activity, like those below, that's expressly for the purpose of making you laugh. Laughter should not simply occur by chance and by windfall; laughter can and should occur by design.

- Create opportunities for laughter—bring people together for a casual meal, party, or picnic.
- Especially if you're feeling stressed or overwhelmed, seek out that person with whom you share a sense of humor. Take part in a lighthearted activity, something that would appeal to a child—a trip to the beach, a petting zoo, an amusement park.
- With a group of friends, take part in a sport or game that none of you are experienced or especially proficient at. Laughter is especially healthy when you're laughing at yourself.
- Don't feel guilty about enjoying that ridiculous sitcom that makes you laugh. It's good for your health! Without apologies or excuses, schedule it into your evening.
- With friends, go to see a comedy—a silly, lowbrow film, or better yet, a play. Outdoor performances are ideal. Pack a picnic and go enjoy Shakespeare in the park.
- Plan and carry out a truly elegant (but harmless) practical joke.
- Look for opportunities to play and be spontaneous. Don't assume that everything has to be meticulously planned. Wing it. Take wrong turns and get lost. Misadventures are the richest source of comedy.
- Spend time playing with children—yours or someone else's. Kids find far

more to laugh at in life than we do. Indulging your goofy side is easy when you're with children.

TO CREATE A LAUGHTER-FRIENDLY ENVIRONMENT

At home, use essential oil of orange in an aromatherapy diffuser or on a lightbulb (*before* you turn on the light). Lively, warm oil of orange is associated with joy and cheer and will help lift your mood and encourage levity.

At work, use orange oil as an energizer and to keep your spirit light. Sprinkle a few drops on a handkerchief and inhale deeply three times to snap out of that afternoon doldrum. If your work environment permits, use a diffuser to share the joyful smell of orange with everyone else too.

AUTUMN:

SEASON
OF
TRANSITION

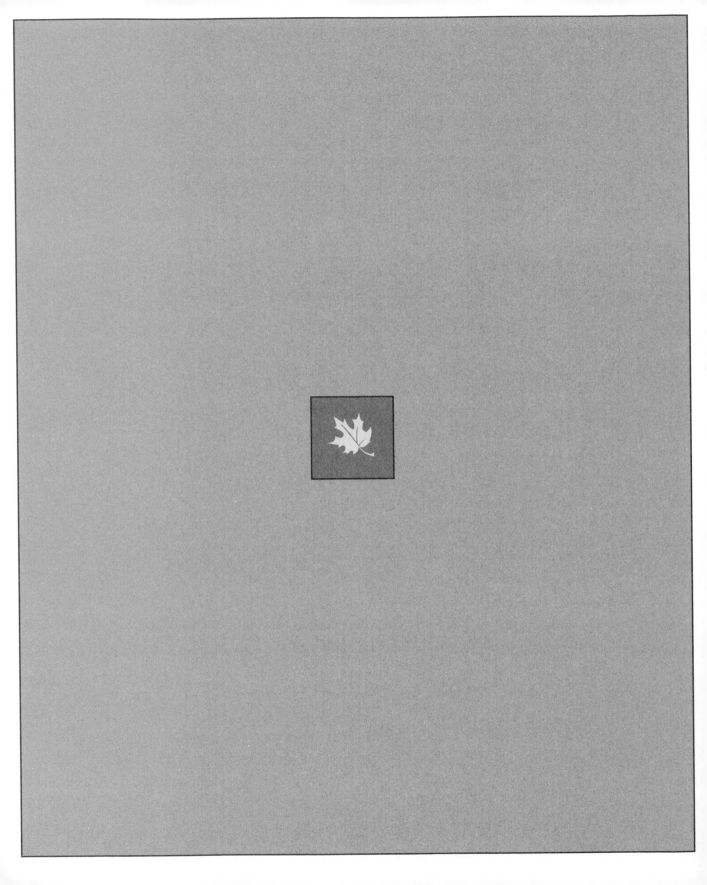

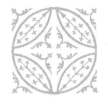

During the dreamy weeks of Indian summer, after the fire energy of the earth finishes its cycle, we revel in the richness of the natural world, the abundant fruits and vegetables. Plants reach maturity, the time when their essential oils are most potent and their fragrance most intense. At this moment, the growth of the summer has mostly ended, though withering and decay have not yet begun. Ripeness, of course, is often just a day away from decay, so this is a brief and magical period of equilibrium, lasting only two or three weeks. Indian summer is even thought of as a "fifth season" in Chinese medicine, as it falls at the halfway point of the Chinese year.

As autumn arrives, the earth's yang energy, which has been expanding throughout spring and summer, changes direction. The cool breath of yin extinguishes the fire element and the natural world turns inward. Now the earth element exerts its influence. Though we may be tempted to resist the "dying of the light" of summer, this new phase is an equally important and necessary part of the life cycle. Like the earth, we need rest in order to rejuvenate. We need to stop and allow life energy to accumulate and build back up. Autumn is the beginning of this vital process.

Our senses register the change of momentum. We feel warmth giving way to coolness. We feel the moisture evaporating from the soil. We hear the autumn wind stir the dry grasses and rattle the leaves. We smell wood smoke as fires are lit in the evenings. Our eyes note the shift in sunlight as it becomes more golden. Indeed, autumn can be dazzling, and in many regions autumn foliage outshines the glory of spring's blossoms. Because of the haze that softens the sky during the fall, autumn sunsets are usually the most brilliant of the year. Autumn is the year's swan song. And perhaps not surprisingly, it's the most difficult season of the year for many people. Instead of welcoming the energetic changes afoot, many of us try to resist.

As the days grow shorter, we may grow anxious. As beautiful as the season's changes are, the death of the year reminds us of our own mortality. As a result, we may find ourselves suffused in a poetic melancholy or struggling in the grip of a bona fide depression. In Chinese medicine, the emotion that symbolizes the season is grief. Grief is not an emotion that we're terribly good at expressing in our culture, because it is usually accompanied by a fear of loss. If we are able to set aside that fear and accept loss as a part of our natural life cycle, grief can be experienced as a beautiful and cleansing emotion. Autumn invites us to make room for this state of mind and enables us to experience its benefits. During this season, the sunset of the year, the beauty and poetry of grief and the release that it offers can enrich our lives.

The harvest season yields wonderful food, and feasts like Thanksgiving remind us of the bounty of the natural world. The energy of plants is now moving down into their roots, and root vegetables help us attune our energy to that of the season. The golden and orange vegetables of autumn, like carrots and sweet potatoes, are rich with beta-carotene, which helps purify and protect our body by fighting free radicals.

The hearth and home should now become our focus as we leave behind summer's adventures and explorations. It is time to withdraw, to close, and to conserve. Instead of eating foods raw, we cook them and preserve them. Traditional seasonal activities like canning and preserving foods from the harvest help us attune ourselves to earth's energy.

The warm colors of the world around us—gold, red, orange, brown—what we think of as "earth tones," are associated with the earth element. The textural quality of materials and surfaces becomes more interesting as we think about preparing our "nest" for the winter. Natural, substantial materials like wood and stone give us the sense of security and warmth we're starting to crave. The desire for change often inspires decorating or remodeling projects in the fall. Just be aware that a decorating project initiated in the fall may have a distinctly different look than one initiated in the spring! As the playful energy of summer fades into memory, we may also find ourselves rededicated to work. Our mood is less frivolous and carefree. We may experience a renewed sense of purpose or focus in our work as we reconnect with our inner mental energies. We begin projects that help us restore order in our home or offices. There is a sense of preparation. Many of us will associate this feeling with "getting ready for the holidays," but it actually harkens back to getting ready for the challenge of surviving winter. This is the season in which our energies should be manifesting themselves in finished products and completed projects. Your mental energy now takes center stage as your physical energy begins to ebb. What may have seemed overwhelming or complicated in the summertime may now reveal itself to you as a straightforward, step-by-step project. Autumn is the easiest time to dazzle your boss or partner with your effectiveness and can-do attitude. It is a great time to take on responsibility—within reason, of course. It's very important not to overload yourself; your body may not yet be up to the challenge of your newly ambitious mind. Conservation of energy is one of the keys to autumn attunement: You should be working smarter, not harder.

In the midst of all this work, we're urged to reproduce. Autumn is the human mating season! A surge of hormones can send our bodies into a tizzy. Your skin may erupt; your temper can grow short. In the Eastern view, this season is a return to the influence of feminine energy, and coupled with our heightened libido, it can be an extraordinarily romantic time. If we are without a mate or lover, we may mourn past relationships or experience sadness over our aloneness.

An ancient Chinese text refers to "rumors of war in the air," an apt metaphor for the seasonal feeling of unease that often accompanies this hormonal cycle, which is further aggravated by our ancient fears about the impending winter. In drier climates, autumn brings the threat of fires and an edge of tension. We are concerned with self-preservation and can easily grow suspicious and agitated. Just like our other major directional change in the spring, we may think we need to make a major change in our life. We may feel brash and aggressive, as if we should take action, grab the bull by the horns, quit that job, dump that boyfriend, or lay down the law with a lazy teenage kid!

Instead, take a deep breath, sit back, and just let the world change around you. Autumn is a true test of our ability to adapt, to respond appropriately. It is a time when communication and appropriate action is highlighted. As our ancestors' communities readied themselves for the challenges of winter, cooperation and interaction were essential. Autumn is a time when calmness and order can provide enormous benefits for our well-being.

THE CHRYSANTHEMUM ALTAR

The color of the season is golden yellow, symbolizing the energy of the earth element. There is still an abundance of color in the flowers of Indian summer, but the colors are richer and deeper. The pastels of spring and summer give way to deeper hues. Gold is ever present.

We are about to enter a new, quieter period of the year, when action is replaced by contemplation, when heat is replaced by coolness, when moisture is replaced by dryness. The sun's rays no longer encourage growth but instead promote drying. Traditional seasonal activities include the drying of grains and fruits to store for use in the winter. While it is a time of preparation, it's also a time of letting go.

This ritual is designed to help you align your energy and expectations with this important seasonal passage. It will help you acknowledge the end of growth and see the beauty and purpose of the next cycle, a cycle of decline that is as essential to life as growth. It is a beautiful and simple way to acknowledge and honor the ability to "let go," which is essential to staying balanced during the autumn.

• Select a place to display your flowers and prepare a small area of sacred space for your bouquet. It should be clean and uncluttered.

• Visit your garden, neighborhood flower stand, or florist. If you are fortunate enough to be growing chrysanthemums or other golden-yellow flowers, then begin your ritual in your own garden. Select a small bouquet of mums, small sunflowers, or other autumn flowers in the golden yellow and brown hues. Look for the ones that have the deepest, most saturated golden quality, even an orange tint.

• Place the vase containing your flowers on inexpensive straw, grass, or wood fiber place mat, ideally one that's thin but loosely woven to permit some air circulation. If you can, choose one that's not dyed or bleached but simply left in the natural color of the materials. Place the vase toward the rear of the mat, leaving a space in front of it.

• After you've enjoyed your flowers for a day, select a particularly beautiful flower and snip it off. Place it on the mat in front of the vase. As you enjoy your bouquet, also observe the transformation taking place in this particular flower: the changes in color, texture, moisture.

• The next day, choose another and repeat the process for the course of about five days. By the time you have five flowers in various states of dryness on the mat, you'll be ready to discard the bouquet.

• If possible, move the mat near a sunny window and let the flowers continue to dry for another five days, or until the petals become crisp.

• Finally, pull the dry petals from the flowers and place them in a small decorative bowl. As you do, note the slightly sharp, spicy scent that still rises from them and be aware of the texture of their dried petals. Keep this bowl on one of your household altars.

• When the first windy day of autumn arrives, sit for a simple meditation, asking yourself before you do to discover something about your life that you would like to release or let go of. This doesn't have to be a negative trait or behavior; it could include an idea, a person, a place, or a material object you've had a difficult time giving up.

• During your meditation, allow yourself to experience the emotion that is stirred by this idea, person, place, or object. As you do, envision that emotion pouring out of you, melting into the bowl of golden flower petals, and infusing them with its energy. Afterward, direct your attention briefly to the empty place where the feeling had been.

• Now carry your bowl outside. Take a whiff of the scent of the dried flower petals and then scatter them into the air and let them blow away, carrying away whatever you wanted to release.

RELIEF *for* TIRED EYES

Caution: Do not perform any foot massage if you are pregnant. Do not perform any massage of the legs if you have varicose veins or blood clots.

These days many of us work under fluorescent lights in our offices, schools, hospitals, and stores. The "strobing," or flickering, of fluorescent lights can be agitating, and the wavelengths of light emitted by fluorescent fixtures are limited, making the colors around us appear washed out and sickly. Other sources of eyestrain and fatigue are the television and computer, both fixtures in the daily lives of many of us. Even if we don't use a computer at work, we're spending more and more time on computers at home. Our visual sense corresponds with the fire element, and the relentless light of a video screen creates a buildup of "heat" in the eyes, producing a burning, dry feeling. Many of us switch off a computer when we leave work, only to flip on a television to unwind when we get home.

During the fall, there's usually an increase in air pollution, making it an even more difficult season for our eyes. On top of that, any emotion that intensifies fire increases eyestrain. If you're stressed or upset, your eyes will be affected. When our eyes are tired and sore, our window on the world becomes painful to look through. Because the visual sense is such a strong one, this can have an unexpectedly dramatic impact on our sense of well-being and our overall mood. Cooling your entire system helps relieve excess heat in the eyes. The best way to rest the eyes is to close them, whether through meditation or sleep. But this next ritual, inspired by Tibetan Ayurveda, is a unique alternative approach to treating overtired, overheated eyes. It is perfect for those who have a hard time tearing themselves away from their computer, yet it works by stimulating reflex points on the feet to draw the heat out of the eyes.

2 bath towels

1 tablespoon of butter or ghee at room temperature

1 tablespoon ground anise

2 small bowls for butter and anise

2 smooth, flat stones, about 6 in. long

(or Body and Soul Stones, see Resources)

Heavy pan or kettle with a tight-fitting lid filled with hot water

for warming stones

A footbath, large shallow bowl, or dish tub filled with

very warm water

6 drops lavender essential oil

1 thermal pitcher of hot but not scalding water

(if your footbath is not self-warming)

Peppermint tea

1 small soft towel

A footstool, low table, or ottoman

1 hand towel

A pair of soft cotton socks

Eye pillow or moist washcloth

• Select a comfortable armchair that allows you to sit with your feet flat on the floor. Place one bath towel on the floor in front of the chair; you'll need to protect the floor from splashes from the footbath. Put butter or ghee and anise powder each in a small bowl. Put your stones into a saucepan of hot water and cover to keep them as warm as possible. Place your supplies where you can reach them easily from the chair; a small side table is ideal. Dim the lights.

• Fill the footbath with very warm water and add the 6 drops of lavender oil. Slip your feet into the warm water and relax for about ten minutes, keeping your eyes closed as much as possible. Add hot water from the thermal pitcher if your footbath cools. Sip your peppermint tea.

• Take your feet out of the water and gently blot them dry with the small soft towel. Move the footbath out of the way and replace with the low table, ottoman, or footstool. Cover it with the bath towel from the floor. Cover your lap with the other bath towel.

The feet contain reflex points for the entire body. Reflex points for the head are located on and below the toes. The eye reflexes can be located at the base of the little toes; you'll feel a little ridge there, formed by the metatarsal joints.

• Bring your right foot up onto your lap, grasping it firmly in your right hand. Using your right hand, pull the fleshy pad under the toes down to access the reflex points for the eyes. Using firm but gentle pressure, "walk" your left thumb along the ridge beneath the toes, focusing on the area beneath the little toe. Stay conscious of your breathing; as you press the reflex point, exhale fully, encouraging your body to relax. Repeat this sequence six times.

• Now move to the head and sinus reflexes. Support the toes with your right hand and use the left thumb to gently press and "walk" your way down from the tip of the big toe to the base. Switch directions when you reach the little toe and repeat the manipulations on each toe.

• Repeat the massage sequence on the left foot, using your left hand to support it and your right hand to massage.

• Dip into the now-softened butter or ghee and massage a small amount into your feet. Then dip your fingers into the anise and apply the herb generously over the left foot. Massage the foot lightly but vigorously for two minutes with the entire palm of your hand. The gritty sensation should feel good—stimulating and relaxing at once. Repeat this on the right foot, making sure the feet are well coated with the anise. Take several deep breaths of the aroma of this herb.

• Taking your hand towel, fold it in half and roll it into a tube. Holding it over the footbath, pour the hot water from your thermal pitcher into it.

- Using caution to prevent yourself from being scalded, squeeze out the hand towel. Wrap your feet in the warm towel, put them up on the footstool or ottoman, and wrap the bath towel around it to retain as much heat as possible. Once again, close your eyes and relax.

- Before the hot towel cools, unwrap your feet and use the towel to remove the herbs. You can use a bit more of the hot water from your pitcher to help cleanse. Your feet will still be a bit oily from the butter.

- Take the warm stones out of the heating pan (be careful; the water may still be quite hot) and blot them dry briefly on the towel. Position the stones on the footstool or ottoman in a position that enables you to place the soles of your feet on them, with your legs at a 45-degree angle. (The Body and Soul Stones have special stimulating bumps that you can position over the eye reflex points.) Relax and enjoy some more tea for at least another five minutes. (Peppermint helps cool the fire element.) The earth element manifested in the stones is wonderfully grounding and helpful for settling down a racing mind.

- Now put on soft cotton socks and lie down on a sofa or bed, covering your eyes with an eye pillow or a moist washcloth. Enjoy your refreshed, soothed eyes and a new sense of calm!

ANXIETY-EASING MUD TREATMENT

The autumn transition is a difficult one because the expanding energy of the spring and summer is now reversing its direction. As we've discussed, this reminds us of our own mortality and vulnerability.

Though the earth element rules autumn, both the seasonal transitions of autumn and spring will feel the influence of air, which is present whenever change is afoot. The winds of autumn are different from the fresh breezes of spring, however—they are not stirring the earth to life but presiding over the drying and desiccation of plants. These winds fill the air with negative ions, causing our tempers to flare, amplifying small irritations, and intensifying anxiety.

One of my clients described the sensation she feels during this time of year as being "emotionally raw, like an oyster out of its shell." Remember, this vulnerability is not necessarily a negative state. The energy shift that is taking place is restoring feminine energy, and that means we are actually growing more receptive to change and new ideas. Still, we feel deprived of the power and confidence that filled us during spring and summer and think that losing it may put us at risk. We may attempt to take control in sporadic bursts, becoming strangely impulsive. This is a time when many relationships are suddenly on the rocks for no apparent reason. Being aware of this seasonal pattern can save you a lot of heartache!

If you visit the Ojai Valley Inn and Spa in Ojai, California, you can experience a native Californian treatment called the *kuyam*. One of the reasons this treatment is so wonderful is that it's a self-treatment, a sort of mud "lodge" where people relax in a communal setting and slather themselves with rich local clay. This similar treatment uses materials from the earth—clay, honey, cornmeal, and natural oil to exert a "grounding" effect and ease the symptoms of nervous tension, anxiety, and even panic attacks. Clay has marvelous exfoliating properties. Many people don't realize that clay dissolves dead skin cells beautifully and is much gentler on the skin than harsh abrasives. Cornmeal is a fairly soft exfoliant that is well suited to treating the body. Honey has hydrating benefits and has been used since ancient times in skin treatments. The nutrients and live enzymes of the fresh carrots are a simple, natural way to detoxify and awaken the skin. Carrot oil, being a root oil, is the opposite of the leaf oils, which affect the mental energies—it is a *deep* oil that is grounding and anchoring and restores our connection with our physical energies. Used for centuries to soothe and heal, chamomile is one of the most calming essential oils, applied topically or inhaled. Because of the Body-Mind connection, we can treat anxiety (a subtle-body problem) on the physical body, using our sense of touch.

This simple mud treatment has three phases, so be sure to read the instructions all the way through before beginning.

YOU WILL NEED:

Space heater or heat lamp if needed

1 cup bentonite clay (available at many natural foods stores and sometimes sold in bulk at herbalists. If you know of a source of pure, nontoxic local clay, it's much better to use that, as local materials will "attune" you more effectively)

¹/₃ cup honey

2 large carrots, puréed

¹/₃ cup cornmeal

1 bath towel you don't mind getting dirty

A soft natural bristle brush (a body brush is best; see Resources)

1 body brush, or washcloth, or loofah

A small shower stool (optional)

2 tablespoons hazelnut oil

6 drops carrot seed oil (optional)

6 drops roman chamomile essential oil (optional)

• Turn up the heat, or use a small space heater to warm your bathroom. It's important to stay warm during this process.

• Mix together the bentonite, honey, carrot purée, and cornmeal in a plastic bowl. Slowly add very hot water until you have created a thick but spreadable batter. The mixture will cool somewhat while you perform the next step. Place a towel over it to prevent heat from escaping. It's best not to heat the mixture in a microwave because it can alter the subtle properties of the ingredients.

• Undress completely. Standing on the bath towel, use the natural bristle brush to vigorously brush the skin of the arms and legs, always working toward the heart. This exfoliates dead skin cells and stimulates blood circulation. If your skin is very sensitive or inflames easily, be sure to use lighter pressure.

DETOXIFYING PHASE

• Be sure to test the temperature of the clay mixture before beginning. Take a generous handful of the clay mixture and slather it over your legs, massaging vigorously without grinding the granules of the cornmeal into the skin. Mechanical exfoliants are really most effective when used as a polish, with minimal pressure but lots of movement. Work your way up the body, covering your torso and making sure you thoroughly coat your backside too.

• Inhale deeply as you proceed, and enjoy the fresh, earthy smell. Use both hands to work the mixture into the skin. Continue applying the mud until your entire body is covered. It will begin to dry quickly. Don't scrub your facial skin, and keep the mud on it moist by applying additional layers. If your skin is dry, avoid your face altogether.

• Your skin's detoxification response is triggered by the *weight* of the mud on it as well as the chemistry of the mud. The heavier the layer on the skin, the stronger the skin's "purge" response as it attempts to neutralize the foreign substance on its surface. The oil glands are flushed out and blood circulation increases. If you have a problem with clogged pores or breakouts on your chest or shoulders, this is a great remedy.

• When the mud is damp-dry to the touch but not dried out and cracking, turn on a hot shower. Bring your body brush, washcloth, or loofah. Ideally, you should be seated for this step, so use a shower stool if you have one. Using the brush, slowly work up the legs and arms toward the body. The brush will soften and loosen the clay and let it rinse away. This step is not meant to be vigorous; slow down the pace of the treatment as you go into the relaxation phase.

RELAXATION PHASE

• When you've removed all the clay, blot dry lightly with a towel but leave your skin quite damp. Pour the hazelnut oil into your hand to warm it and add the other oils if you have them. You may want to heat the hazelnut oil (the beaker of a small electric coffeepot works best), but always test the temperature first. The delicious smell of this elegant nut oil, which has a particular affinity for the skin, is seasonally attuning for autumn, when nuts are harvested. Pure carrot seed oil, available in the aromatherapy section of your natural foods store, is deeply nourishing and calming for the skin and contains the antioxidant beta-carotene, which neutralizes free radicals.

• Slowly massage the oil into your skin with medium-pressure effleurage strokes, always working toward the heart. It will seal moisture in the skin and nourish it. A generous and gentle oiling of the body, using firm pressure with the full palm of the hand, has a magical effect on nervous anxiety. For a different result, try using a technique from another native massage modality, Lomi Lomi, the "massage hula" of Hawaii. Lomi uses much more oil than a typical Swedish massage, and the therapist works on you with the broad planes of her forearms. Use your forearms as well as your hands in this self massage, and really try to take your time with this finishing step.

• Conclude with a shower or a bath to remove the excess oil. Use a very gentle cleanser, and don't worry about getting yourself "squeaky clean." Your skin will still have a lovely sheen from the treatment and a moist, healthy texture.

AUTUMN HOUSEKEEPING

This day is designed to cleanse and prepare you for the seasonal transition ahead. Moments of directional change, such as the transition from summer to fall and the transition from winter to spring, are times of vulnerability. You can end up feeling run-down or catching cold easily. The slight chill that you feel in the air at night, even following a hot day, a familiar yet not quite recognizable smell of autumn that wafts by on a little breeze—these are cues. When fall clothes in the stores *finally* pique our interest, it's because earth energy is on the rise. Earth inspires our instinct to enfold, protect, layer, and wrap. Even the vegetables associated with the earth element, such as onions and cabbage, are layered or "wrapped" around a core.

Take advantage of this vital juncture to cleanse and prepare yourself for the shift to the more feminine energy of the autumn and winter. Set aside a morning or afternoon to ready your nest for the winter ahead. The activities of "closing and storing" are inherent to fall. Many of us are much more inspired to clean and organize during the fall than during the traditional "spring" cleaning—even better, since so many chores get neglected during the busy, playful season of summer.

• Begin by cleaning your kitchen, bath, and bedroom, ridding them of any clutter. Environmental congestion reflects inner congestion. Clutter and heaps of debris on your desk or bedside table are often a sign of excessive earth energy, which weighs you down. Old magazines and other outdated reading you haven't gotten around to should be recycled, because they keep you tied to the past. Papers, like the leaves of autumn, have a tendency to pile up in drifts. Rake them up, file them, recycle them. If you live in a small environment and don't have room to put everything away and out of sight, an attractive folding screen can be a practical and effective way to create a serene backdrop. Simplify, refine, and purify your visual environment.

• Launder your bed linens. Spray them lightly with an aromatherapy mist (recipe follows) as you're remaking the bed. Essential oil of cinnamon is a very pleasing essence in environmental applications, though it's not suggested for topical skin care use. Its rich, spicy, and warm smell blends well with the sweetness of vanilla and mandarin orange.

• Instead of discarding your old clothes, books, and personal items, consider donating them to a Salvation Army or women's shelter near you. You attune yourself to the nurturing autumn energy of earth when you donate possessions to someone in need.

Aromatherapy Linen Mist

This is a simple aromatherapy recipe that helps to attune you to autumn's earth energy. These essences, which are also found in some of the season's best-loved desserts, nourish the soul with their sweetness and warmth. It's best to make small batches of aromatherapy mists to ensure their freshness. You can use this wonderful-smelling mist as a room or linen spray.

To two ounces of distilled water, add:
Three drops vanilla essential oil
Three drops cinnamon essential oil
Two drops mandarin orange essential oil

Place in a colored glass (cobalt, amber, or deep green) spray bottle. Shake it well before spraying to disperse the oils in the water. Most plastic breaks down when it comes in contact with essential oils, requiring that you replace the spray pump frequently.

THE CENTER *of the* YEAR

Indian summer is a pause in the energetic momentum of the year, just as meditation is a pause in our mental and physical activity. This brief and dreamy period, with its quality of time suspended, can be especially conducive to meditation. If we're in balance, our Body-Mind will be immersed in Indian summer's atmosphere of peace and plenty. If we are aligned with the energy of the season, we will meld with the feeling of relaxation and ease. It is not yet time for action and preparation for the rigors of winter. Instead, it's an opportunity to step back and savor the abundance of the ripe world around us.

Still, many of us find it difficult to relax. Our bodies may be living in the present but our minds are already racing, anticipating the forthcoming seasonal changes. To be centered, Body and Mind have to be in the same place and existing in the present tense. The following ritual is designed to center you, to bring Body and Mind back together. Meditation is one of the most important healing modalities for any season, but the energetic "center" of the year provides us with a unique opportunity to accept its gifts.

This simple meditation and breathwork ritual takes place outdoors. First, select or create a sacred space for your meditation. If you can, seat yourself at the center of a round or rounded shape. You can look for the shape in nature; a round patch of shade under a tree is perfect. For this ritual, being close to the earth is important; ideally, you should sit on the ground to meditate. This "grounds" you both literally and figuratively.

• Get comfortable and close your eyes. Take three deep breaths into your belly, inhaling to a count of three, exhaling to a count of six. Allow yourself to pause briefly after each inhalation to experience the sensation of your lungs fully expanded. This moment between inhalation and exhalation is symbolic of the season of Indian summer, the pause between growth and decline. It is a wonderful, brief moment that floods your body with a sense of well-being and relaxation. As you pause here with your lungs full, centered, and still, acknowledge the shifting force of the season that is about to lead you in another direction.

• Now, releasing your breath, feel the lungs grow smaller and softer. Feel the inward movement. Go inside to this empty space and try to fully experience it. Don't hurry to fill it with another breath. Once again you are poised between positive and negative, exhalation and inhalation, in a fragile moment of equilibrium few of us ever notice.

• Inhaling again, bring your sensory awareness to the temperature of the warm air, the sound of birds, the smells of the outdoors—soil, plants, and flowers. This is the time of year that vegetation has reached maturity, and plants are releasing lots of their essential oils into the air. Let yourself simply become part of the environment, allowing the sensory experience to flow into you. The empty space inside you becomes a vessel, welcoming the nectar of the senses. The earth element of autumn is embodied by anything that encloses or shelters, such as vessels.

• As you breathe, feel the earth under you and visualize yourself being firmly rooted in it, like the plants around you. Experience the stability and firmness of this solid, enduring base. Feel the earth sheltering you and supporting you.

Feel yourself enfolded in it even as you enfold its sounds, smells, and sensations inside yourself.

• Repeat to yourself the affirmation *There is no effort necessary. I am here.* Begin by speaking it out loud in a relaxed, easy tone of voice. When you repeat it again, do so more quietly, and let your voice fade away until the affirmation is simply inside your head. You don't need to count your repetitions or time yourself; simply repeat the affirmation for a couple of minutes until it quietly disappears.

• Continue to breathe fully but without effort. Repeat the affirmation *I am here. I am at the center. I am safe.* Begin, again, by saying it aloud and then gradually reducing the volume of your voice to a whisper, finally letting it fade away completely.

• After about ten minutes have passed—don't time it—direct your attention back to your senses, to sound and smell and the solid feeling of the earth under you. Gradually open your eyes. Conclude your meditation with a deep inhalation and finally, *smile* as you exhale. Feel the warmth flow from the muscles of your face throughout your body. Enjoy the sense of peacefulness and well-being.

THE AUTUMN LOVE FEAST

With autumn's harvest, the earth is sharing her bounty. Have you noticed your appetite increasing as the temperature drops? This is an ancient physiological response that helps us prepare for the cold months ahead. We can now moderately increase our caloric intake, focusing on richer tissue-building proteins and complex carbohydrates from whole grains. The light, low-fat fruits and vegetables of summer don't provide us with the warmth and substance we need now. Beans, sprouted grains, and nuts are protein-rich seasonal produce. Beware of the empty carbohydrates (and sugars) that pass for "fat-free foods"—they will excite air energy, which can increase autumnal nervousness and anxiety.

In food, autumn's yellow and orange color signals the presence of beta-carotene, which turns into vitamin A in the body. Beta-carotene is essential for the metabolism of protein and gives a boost to our immune system, which is important for preparing our bodies for the onslaught of the flu season. Dark greens like spinach, chard, beet greens, and kale are also in season and are an excellent source of beta-carotene.

Autumn is the season of feasting, and as we've discussed, our attitude and intentions when eating are vitally important to the energy the food provides for our Body-Mind. A number of researchers have investigated the ability of humans to affect the biochemistry of food with their thoughts. One such investigator is physician Leonard Laskow, author of the book *Healing with Love*, whose signature experiment transforms the flavor of wine with "loving intention."

Our practice of praying over our food once it has been placed on the table suggests that our ancestors understood that directing loving thoughts and gratitude toward our meal, which symbolized God's grace, would make it even more beneficial for us. Even if you are not in the practice of saying grace with a meal, simply pausing and offering your silent, heartfelt gratitude will help you benefit more fully from the food you eat. And offering thanks for your meals may even inspire you to make better choices; it's harder to imagine grace embodied by left-over pizza, for example.

This ritual can be performed with an entire meal or with a single food or beverage. Beverages are perhaps the easiest to use. Whatever you pick, just make sure that you have enough to divide what you have prepared into two containers and to provide everyone present with a serving. It can be done alone, but in the spirit of seasonal attunement, it is a lovely ritual for a party or family gathering.

A beverage of your choice
2 identical containers or flasks for your chosen beverage
2 glasses for each person present, ideally identical

• Divide the beverage into the two identical containers and mark the bottom of one with a little heart.

• Take the unmarked flask into another room for the duration of the love infusion.

• Have everyone present close their eyes. Then ask everyone to simply quiet and calm themselves with about six deep breaths. This gives some time for the nervous laughter and jokes to subside, and it helps everyone to center themselves.

• Tell your group, "We are going to use our shared, loving intentions to transform this beverage into a healing elixir." Have everyone visualize a glowing golden light surrounding their entire body, radiating outward and filling the room. After a moment, ask them to envision this light concentrating its brightness and power in their hands.

• Tell them that as the flask is passed around from person to person, to infuse this glowing energy into the liquid it contains. They can silently express their gratitude for the beverage. (Dr. Laskow is said to thank the grape growers and grape pickers and winemakers who created the wine he uses in his demonstration.) They can direct loving intention toward it, asking that it be transformed into an elixir that will bring happiness and well-being to everyone who drinks it.

• Pass the flask around, ensuring that everyone have a moment or two with it. Then set it aside with the untreated flask and allow it, in Laskow's words, to "restructure" for about ten to fifteen minutes.

• Give everyone two glasses, and mark them to indicate which contains treated and untreated liquid. Decant both liquids, and compare the flavors of the beverages. Most people find that the flavor of the treated liquid has been transformed. Depending on the beverage used, it may taste sweeter, softer, richer, or more pleasant. When wine is treated, it seems to be less tannic and sharp. Tap water tastes more pure.

• Ask everyone to drink their entire "treated" sample. If you're using wine, make sure you use a very small amount, perhaps a half glass, so that the effects of the alcohol will not be significant.

• Note the changes in your group after about thirty minutes. Most people find that their group experiences an upswelling of distinct positive energy. The discussion that's stimulated by this ritual may set a wonderful new precedent for holiday dinner table conversation.

This ritual underscores the importance of treating even seemingly mundane daily activities like eating and drinking as a means of enhancing your well-being and happiness. After you perform it, you'll probably look at meals very differently!

AROMATHERAPY *for* HEALTHY LUNGS

The lungs are the system of the body highlighted in autumn, the time of the year when we encounter our first bout of colds and flu. The change of direction that takes place in the earth's energy during autumn brings with it greater risk of illness and emotional upset. The destabilizing influence of air is present during seasonal changes; we feel it in the breezes and see it scattering dead leaves in the street. We may feel it in our own uneasiness or irritability. While Western physicians may scoff at the idea of a draft or dampness being able to cause a cold, even your grandma agreed with traditional Chinese medicine on this point. Protect your lungs during this season by assiduously avoiding cold drafts and cold, damp conditions. When you're outdoors, even if you're warmed up, it's a good idea to protect the neck, particularly the back of the neck, by wearing a turtleneck or a scarf. If you've perspired during your workout, quickly change out of your damp exercise clothes and take a hot shower. Don't allow yourself to get chilled.

In Chinese medicine the lungs are considered the source of immune energy, or *wei chi*. The lungs bring the outside world into our body with each breath we take, nourishing and enlivening our body with oxygen. They are known as the Tender Organ, because as they oversee the interface between the inner and outer world, they are exposed to the dangers of the latter. As we've discussed, autumn is a point of contact between the inner (yin) and outer (yang) world and the cycle of breathing is a perfect representation of this duality. Yang is visible in inhalation, with its expansion and absorption of oxygen's life energy. Yin is expressed in exhalation, with its contraction and release of waste. This simple aromatherapy ritual will help ensure that your lungs stay healthy and strong during this time of change.

Respiration Blend

Caution: This blend is not for topical use. If you get essential oils on your hands during preparation, wash them thoroughly with soap and water. Do not apply to the skin and use caution to make sure that you do not get any essential oils in your eyes.

6 drops eucalyptus essential oil
3 drops peppermint essential oil
6 drops fir essential oil

3 drops pine essential oil
6 drops lavender essential oil
1 tablespoon squalane or jojoba oil
An aromatherapy diffuser, a pan of warm water
on the stove, or a small electric drip coffeemaker,
switched to on, with the beaker full of hot water

• Put the drops of essential oil into the carrier oil and mix them together. The carrier will help prevent them from evaporating as quickly. Pour the mixture into your chosen diffuser, pan, or beaker. After a few minutes, this refreshing blend of essential oils will begin to permeate the room. This is a good blend to use as a preventive whenever there are colds in the household. As soon as you can smell them, you know that the aromatic essences have started their good work.

• Sit quietly in a chair for a few minutes and gently direct your attention to your breath. When you have focused, inhale on a count of six, filling your lungs from top to bottom. Exhale on a slow count of three. Repeat five times or until you experience a sensation of relaxation and calm.

• For your safety, make sure you extinguish a candle diffuser and turn off any electrical diffuser or heating source. Set a timer for 30 to 60 minutes to remind you.

AFTER-WORK AROMATHERAPY

Autumn refocuses our energy from outside to inside, from physical activity to mental activity. If we're experiencing a lot of stress and find ourselves out of balance, we may end our day feeling weak, fatigued, or depressed. As night falls, the fire energy that still brightens autumn's skies fades away, and we may find our energy fading along with it. When you understand what is happening during this energy shift, you'll be mentally prepared and probably find the transition markedly easier. Because the sense of smell is so acute during this season, you'll find that aromatherapy rituals are particularly effective for creating Body-Mind balance.

This after-work aromatherapy "cocktail" for the body contains essential oils known for their ability to uplift and energize. This is a wonderful ritual to perform if you'd like a quick but profound restorative after a long day—a good substitute for zoning out in front of the television or having a glass of wine to unwind. Bergamot, a citrusy perfumer's oil that is included in many men's and women's fragrances, has marvelous uplifting and refreshing properties. Clary sage is a euphoric and highly effective against depression and nervous tension. It's recommended that you not drive after using clary sage, in fact, so you may want to reserve this ritual for after you're settled in for the evening. Thyme strengthens at many levels—physical, emotional, and mental—making it an especially attuning oil for autumn. It stimulates the brain, easing fatigue as well as anxiety. Rosemary is a nervous-system stimulant that improves mental clarity and relieves nervous and emotional exhaustion.

Caution: Do not use this blend if you are pregnant. Do not apply this blend before sun exposure. Bergamot in particular will make you extra sensitive to ultraviolet light and can cause darkening of the skin. Always perform a patch test whenever trying a new essential oil.

YOU WILL NEED:
16 drops bergamot essential oil
8 drops clary sage essential oil
4 drops thyme essential oil
4 drops rosemary essential oil

*2 ounces unscented body oil or lotion for aromatherapy
blending (see Resources)*

• Begin with a shower to wash away the cares of the day and clear the mind.

• Combine essential oils with lotion or body oil. This recipe will yield about four applications for a generous massage.

• Seat yourself in a quiet, warm, comfortable, and private spot. Massage the aromatic blend gently over the entire body. When massaging the arms and legs, work upward toward the heart. When massaging the abdomen, use light pressure and clockwise strokes. Take your time and enjoy the sensation of healing touch.

• In your refreshed and relaxed state, prepare and enjoy a seasonally attuning supper.

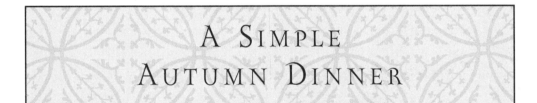

A SIMPLE AUTUMN DINNER

After eating lots of raw foods during the summer, which are cooling, it's time to create inner warmth by cooking what we eat. The return to the heart of our home, the kitchen, is a happy one. Your sense of smell is highlighted during autumn, making food preparation and eating more enjoyable. This is nature's way of ensuring that our appetite will be whetted and that we'll increase our caloric intake, preparing us for the cold weather ahead.

This rich-tasting vegetarian soup is the perfect way to welcome fall. It includes some of the season's root vegetables, to help attune you to earth energy, as well as mushrooms, one of autumns treasures. The croutons are the perfect accompaniment.

Forest Soup with Roasted Garlic Croutons

FOR THE SOUP:

1/2 pound fresh shiitake, chanterelle, or morel mushrooms

(preferably locally foraged or grown) cut into large pieces

1 1/2 tablespoons ghee

1 yellow onion chopped into 1/2-inch pieces

1/3 cup dry white wine

1 cup organic barley

2 quarts water

1 red bell pepper

1 clove garlic, minced

4 carrots, peeled and diced

2 parsnips, peeled and diced

2 stalks of celery, diced

3 fresh sage leaves

1/4 cup fresh thyme sprigs

1 teaspoon sea salt

Fresh cracked pepper to taste

FOR THE CROUTONS:

1 head of garlic

2 tablespoons extra virgin olive oil

Fresh baked whole-grain bread sliced into 2-inch squares

1. Wash and remove woody stems from the mushrooms and cut them lengthwise into large pieces. Melt ghee in a soup pot and add onion, sautéing it until it has caramelized. Be sure to stir it frequently to prevent it from burning. Deglaze the pot with the wine and add the mushrooms

and barley, stirring them for 5 minutes before adding the rest of the ingredients. Simmer, covered, for 90 minutes.

2. While the soup is cooking, prepare croutons. Cut off the top of a head of garlic, douse the cloves with a tablespoon of olive oil, wrap in foil, and bake at 375 degrees for an hour. After it cools slightly, squeeze the now-caramelized garlic out of the head into a small bowl. Whisk with a tablespoon of olive oil to create a creamy spread. You can prepare roasted garlic in advance and keep it on hand as a warming, immune-boosting condiment.

3. Immediately before the soup is done cooking, lightly brush both sides of the bread squares with olive oil and toast them on a cookie sheet at 400 degrees, turning them once. Remove after 4 minutes and spread with the roasted garlic blend.

4. Remove the thyme sprigs from the soup and ladle into heated bowls. Float two or three croutons in each bowl and enjoy!

DEVELOPING STRENGTH and ROUTINE

Another metaphoric title for the lungs in Chinese medicine is the "Officials of Rhythmic Order." This orderliness is one of the key themes for the most beneficial seasonal fitness activities in autumn. This is not the playful, make-it-up-as-you-go-along season of summer, but a time of thoughtful preparation. Responsibility, pragmatism, and level headedness are traits that ensure you will be aligned with the energy of the season. The fact that autumn is back-to-school season makes perfect sense. With yin energy ascending, we are more obedient now and more willing to listen. We are ready for the rhythmic order of a set daily routine. While we may resist the end of our season of play, an autumn routine often fills us with a deep sense of satisfaction. As a result, autumn is an ideal time to begin a fitness program, because you will be receptive to discipline and routine.

If you are doing rigorous physical training at this time of year, you'll need to schedule more time for rest. You'll need to make sure that you're meditating regularly to keep your inward focus strong. Your diet will need to include even more protein-rich tissue-building foods, since hard training breaks down and rebuilds muscle. It is best to opt for a moderate but steady exercise plan. You'll feel better and stay healthier.

Building strength is one of the keys to autumn fitness, and this is an excellent time to begin a weight-training program. This simple program can quickly enhance muscle tone and strength without adding bulk. You'll see gratifying results within four weeks. You'll also be aware of increased strength as you perform everyday acts like lugging a tote bag, hoisting a suitcase into an overhead bin on an airplane, or scooping up a toddler. Better still, free-weight strength training is easy to do at home and requires a minimum of equipment.

Caution: Do not begin this or any other exercise program before consulting with your physician. If at any time you feel dizzy or nauseated, stop. Stop immediately if you feel any chest pain, unusual pressure in your chest, or if you experience a "cold sweat." Be mindful of any sharp, unusual, or intensifying pain and contact your health-care practitioner. Always squat to lift your weights, never bending from the waist.

YOU WILL NEED:
A set of two- to five-pound dumbbells (adjustable dumbbells
are practical, since you will progress to heavier weights)
A set of ankle weights (begin with about 2 to 6 pounds in each cuff)
A rug or carpeted floor, clear of obstacles

A sturdy chair
Athletic shoes with socks thick enough to protect your ankles
from the weight cuffs
Comfortable, loose-fitting workout clothes
Music that sets a relaxed, upbeat mood but won't goad
you to work too fast

It's important to rest between sets, and there is no reason to hurry this rest period. Remember, activity and rest have equal importance. There is no "right" length of time to rest, but you'll know when it's time to begin another set. You'll feel strong and ready.

This entire program should take only about thirty minutes to complete, and should be performed twice a week.

• Precede your strength training with a warm-up. It can be as simple as five minutes of marching in place, jogging in place, or even dancing to some of your favorite music. The important thing is to get circulation going and to spend at least five minutes on this. When you're done with your warm-up, turn on your training music. Though you can "zone out" and watch TV while you exercise, you'll benefit more if you stay focused on what you're doing. Our tendency to layer too many activities diminishes our ability to derive maximum enjoyment and benefit from each. Repetition can be dull or it can be meditative. Let your routine lull you into a relaxed but alert "flow" state. Many women report doing their most creative thinking while exercising.

• Begin your strength training with this awareness exercise, to center you. It's important that you be focused and centered, with your abdominal muscles contracted, when working with even the lightest weights. The lower back in particular is very fragile. This simple floor sequence takes some of its inspiration from The Method, a wonderful form of exercise based on the teaching of Joseph Pilates that builds strength and flexibility simultaneously. Originally designed to rehabilitate injured dancers, The Method has been around for years but has recently attained newfound popularity among entertainers and athletes. The smoothness and grace of the exercise makes it a true pleasure—more akin to doing yoga than lifting weights. Specially trained and certified instructors are required to master this fascinating discipline. (See Resources.) Two of its key principles are the strengthening of the girdle of muscles that supports the lower back and abdomen and the dynamic use of breath in every exercise.

ABDOMINAL SEQUENCE

• Lie on the floor with your arms at your sides, knees bent. Breathe in a relaxed manner through your nose for about half a minute. Now inhale through your nose and exhale through your mouth with a soft "shhhhhhh!" sound. Doing this helps to control and lengthen the exhalation, supporting your exertion through the entire range of motion. As you exhale, contract your abdominal muscles and press your lower back to the floor. As you inhale, release the contraction and let your spine come up off the floor, shifting your weight gently toward the tailbone in a smooth movement. Repeat this six times. This is an excellent movement for loosening the lower back. You can use it between these or any abdominal exercises for a nice release.

• Place your hands lightly behind your head. Take a deep breath through your nose, and as you exhale, press your lower back to the floor and lift your head, neck, and shoulders without straining, in a subtle abdominal "crunch." Do not pull on your head and neck with your hands, and don't jerk your body forward. The movement should be very smooth and gentle. Focus on your contracted abdominal muscles and keeping your lower back in contact with the floor. You don't need to come up very far at all to feel this exercise. Inhaling, smoothly ease back down to the floor. Repeat this twenty times, then lie flat for a moment and make yourself aware of the warming sensation in your abdominal muscles.

• Now, lying on your back, raise your feet into the air, straightening your legs without making them rigid. With your arms at your sides, gently inscribe a little circle in the air with your feet, exhaling with the effort. After a quick inhale, reverse the direction, making another circle and exhaling again. The rhythm should be steady but not fast. You should hear your breath in a rhythmic "shhh! shhh! shhh! shhh!" The more control you exert over your feet, the harder your abdominal muscles will work. Try expanding the size of your circles and then reducing them until they are very small. Repeat twenty times.

• Once again place your hands behind your neck lightly—don't pull upward—exhale, and raising yourself up, touch your right elbow to your left knee. As you do so, extend your right leg, pointing the toe. Now switch, initiating a slow-motion "pedaling" movement. Continue to exhale firmly with short, sharp "shhh!" sounds, focusing on keeping your lower back pressed to the floor. Repeat twenty times. Finish with the original spinal-loosening sequence, about six times. When you're done, lie still for a moment.

• Roll over onto your hands and knees to do a simple "cat" stretch. Inhaling and lowering your head to look back at your legs, arch your back up like a cat; then reverse the motion, bowing your belly down toward the floor, lifting your chin and extending outward from your tailbone. Repeat this six times.

You need very little weight to build strength. If you stay focused and move slowly, even light weights can create excellent results in firming and building muscle. This program will be quite effective with just two sessions per week. The first week of your strength-training routine will be a "get-acquainted" period, when you discover how much weight you need. You can determine this by increasing weight incrementally until you find the point at which you are feeling significant exertion, even a bit of muscle trembling, at ten repetitions. If you've done weight training and are accustomed to doing more repetitions at higher weights, remember that the slow, deliberate movement and careful control of the reverse movement significantly increase the exertion required.

LOWER BODY ROUTINE

Caution: When you put on your ankle weights, be careful; you don't have the same balance and mobility you normally do. They can get caught on each other and trip you as well. Move slowly and deliberately whenever you're wearing ankle weights. Don't walk around in ankle weights; this can strain the knees.

Hamstrings: Attach your ankle weights. If this is the first time you're using them, begin with just one pound in the cuff. This will help you gauge your current level of strength. Stand behind a chair, holding the back, and bend forward from the waist until you are at a forty-five-degree angle. Your feet should be about eighteen inches from the back of the chair, and your upper body, from the tailbone to the top of your head, should form a straight line. Do not lock your knees, but be sure to tighten your abdominal muscles. Inhale through the nose, exhale with a "shhhh!" through your mouth, and bending your right knee, lift your foot back toward yourself as far as it will go. Concentrate on controlling the movement upward and downward. Repeat with your left leg, and complete fifteen repetitions, if possible. Complete two more sets with rests of one minute in between.

Hip extensions: From this same position, you can smoothly segue into hip extensions. Check to make sure your abdominal muscles are still tightened to support your lower back, and also that your left knee is not locked. Exhaling, lift your right leg behind you in a smooth, straight line. Lower your leg at the same slow pace back to the straight position. Switch legs and repeat ten times.

Complete three sets. Your upper thighs and buttocks will be strengthened by this sequence.

Knee extensions: This strengthens your quadriceps, the muscles on the front of the upper thighs. Still wearing your leg weights, sit down on your chair. For this exercise, the seat should be deep enough to support your leg almost to the axis of the knee. Place a rolled-up towel beneath your knees for additional support. Brace yourself lightly by grasping the seat of the chair. Tighten your abdominal muscles, exhale, and then inhale through the nose. Exhaling with a "shhhhh" release of your breath, slowly raise your right leg until it is straight; don't lock your knee at the end of the extension. Inhale through your nose as you lower it at the same speed. Complete three sets of ten to fifteen repetitions.

Hip raise: Still with leg weights on, lie down on your left side, left elbow bent and hand supporting your head, torso facing forward. Exhale, contract your abdominal muscles, and raise your right leg, extending it upward in a line parallel with the body and out through the toe. Inhaling, bring it down with complete control to meet the leg on the floor. Repeat ten to fifteen times. Roll over and repeat the sequence on your right side, lifting and lowering the left leg. Try not to focus on the count but on the sensation of the muscles and on your breath. Make sure your abdominal muscles are engaged to provide support to the lower back. For the next set, lift the leg slightly and extend it, inscribing circles about a foot in diameter with your foot. Return to the original pattern for your third set.

Release: Remove your leg weights. Roll onto your back and grasp your knees to your chest. Gently rock from side to side, just enough to shift the weight from one side of your midback to the other but not enough to roll over. This simple self-massage helps to loosen the back.

Lunges: (*Caution:* Be especially careful or skip this exercise if you have weak knees.) Standing, place your hands on your hips. Exhale, tighten your abdominal muscles, and lunge forward with your right foot about three feet, allowing your left heel to come up and your body to move forward over the right knee. Keep your torso upright, your gaze looking forward, and don't collapse over the lead leg. The right lower leg should be perpendicular to the floor. Push back off the right foot to return to the starting position. Alternate legs and complete three sets of ten full lunges on both legs. If you have the space, you can "walk" forward as you lunge rather than returning to the starting position. To do this, bring the rear leg up toward the forward leg to resume the starting position instead of pushing backward.

After a week of lunges without weights, begin doing your sets with two-pound dumbbells. Increase the weight slowly, as it can destabilize you. Hold the dumbbells by your sides, palms facing inward, and complete the exercise.

Calf raise: This exercise will strengthen the gastrocnemius and soleus muscles. Find a stair or step with secure support from a wall or railing. Make sure you are very stable. The balls of your feet are on the step, with the heels hanging over. Contract your abdominals and make sure your back is not swayed. Inhale through the nose, and exhale, lowering yourself as far as you will comfortably go. Be sure not to overdo it or push yourself if your calves are tight. Inhale again and raise yourself up on your toes. Complete ten repetitions on each foot. When you have finished your reps, lift your foot at the ankle and circle each foot about six times in each direction to loosen it.

UPPER BODY ROUTINE

Biceps: You use your biceps a great deal, and increased strength in this muscle will be a big help in everyday lifting and lugging. You'll feel muscles working in the forearm as well. Pick up a two- to six-pound dumbbell in your right hand. Seat yourself securely on the chair. Sit up straight and contract your abdominal muscles. Don't grip the dumbbell too tightly or your hand may cramp. Allow your right arm to hang straight down at your side. Brace your left hand on your left knee. Exhale and bend your right arm, lifting the dumbbell and pivoting it as it moves upward so that your fingers are facing you when your forearm is upright. Lower the weight slowly back to the starting position. Complete ten repetitions and two to three sets.

Triceps: One of the important concepts behind strength training is to work the anterior and posterior muscles in each area; in this case, work the biceps and the triceps in sequence. This is one of the weakest muscles for women, and when strengthened will firm and tighten the upper arms.

Sitting in a chair, hold a six- to ten-pound dumbbell with both hands and raise it over your head. Turn the dumbbell so that the handle is upright and the inside face of the weight rests on the upturned palms of your hands. Without allowing your elbows to pop out, exhale fully, contract your abdominal muscles, and lift the weight directly over your head. Lower it slowly, and repeat ten times. Complete two sets of this exercise. Squat to put down your weights and rest for a minute.

The final exercise in the triceps sequence is very simple. Stand with feet shoulder-width apart and extend your arms behind you, keeping them close together and as straight as possible. Try not to lean forward. Press arms upward with small pulses as hard as you can for thirty seconds, alternating quick, rhythmic inhalations of three counts with exhalations of three counts. These breaths should match your pulses.

Deltoids: This exercise will firm, define, and strengthen the muscles on the upper outer arms. Stand with your feet shoulder-width apart and contract your abdominal muscles as you exhale. Inhaling, with elbows bent and forearms parallel to the floor, hold two- to six-pound dumbbells upright in front of you. Exhaling, lift your elbows up until they are even with your shoulders, maintaining the ninety-degree angle of your arms as you do. Breathing smoothly and evenly, repeat ten times.

Shoulder row: This will strengthen and develop the biceps, deltoids, and trapezius muscles and stabilize the shoulder joint. Squat to pick up two- to six-pound dumbbells and stand with feet shoulder-width apart, your palms inward. The dumbbells should be resting against your thighs and should be positioned so that they almost touch each other. Inhale through your nose and exhale, lifting the dumbbells straight up while keeping your hands in the same position. Your elbows will move out to the sides and you should finish with your arms parallel to the floor. Pause, inhale, then lower the weights with complete control, exhaling slowly. Repeat ten times and complete two sets.

INCREASING YOUR FLEXIBILITY

Strength benefits us only when it is coupled with flexibility. Flexibility—both physical and mental—is essential to staying balanced and healthy during autumn. Resisting the changes taking place in the inevitable cycle of the seasons puts you at odds with the world around you. Our fear of loss can be triggered by the most innocuous things—the smell of fallen fruit rotting on the ground, the sun-bleached landscape, a dry wind stirring dust. If we are not flexible enough to yield to these seasonal changes, we risk becoming ill or injuring our bodies. This ritual will help you restore resilience in a body that has been made inflexible by stress, overwork, worry, and the illusion of maintaining control over life's events.

The back and shoulders are the parts of the body we associate with work and responsibility. In terms of body mechanics alone, working at a keyboard causes tension and stress in the muscles of the shoulders, especially the trapezius, a large triangle-shaped muscle that extends up the neck and across the shoulders. The vulnerable lower back and lumbar vertebrae are also adversely affected when we sit for long periods of time. This simple Body-Mind fitness stretching ritual can be done anywhere, even in an office cubicle, and brings dramatic relief to strain and tension in the shoulders and neck as well as the lower back.

The first exercise is particularly balancing in autumn because it incorporates the shape of the season in its circular rotation.

HIP ROTATIONS

• Stand at the center of the space you're in. Place your hands flat on the sides of your hips and pretend that a filament is drawing your head upward toward the ceiling.

• Slowly rotate your hips in a smooth circle, clockwise, without collapsing your back or leaning forward. Guide your movement with your hands. Feel the lower spine release; you may even hear a little crack or two. Enjoy the liquid sensation of the rotation at it lubricates your vertebrae.

• To change direction, inscribe a little arabesque with your hips, an "S" shape that you might also envision as the line that divides the symbol for yin/yang.

• Rotate your hips in a counterclockwise direction for a minute, then reverse direction again. A couple of minutes of this gentle rotation will loosen and warm the lower back and provide relief from fatigue caused by sitting.

UPPER BACK, NECK, AND SHOULDER RELEASE

This exercise uses a group of stretches that will work miracles on even rock-hard muscles. Stretches allow blood to flow into muscles that are starved for nourishment. You'll actually feel the soothing warmth of the muscle being irrigated by an infusion of blood after you finish these stretches.

Be sure to share this wonderful ritual with your coworkers. By banishing stubborn muscular tension, you also release emotional tension and help the work environment become more harmonious.

- Stand in the center of your space, feet shoulder-width apart, back straight and head extending toward the ceiling. Extend your arms and cross them at the elbows. Bending them back up toward you, cross them again by bringing the top wrist under the bottom wrist. You may be able to clasp your hands together. Your arms are now entwined.
- Exhaling, very slowly straighten your arms and raise them up as far as you can without straining. When you reach the top, inhale. You'll feel your scapulae (shoulder blades) open.
- Exhaling, lower your arms as far as you can. Feel the stretch through the middle of the trapezius, where it extends across the shoulders.
- Unwind your arms, then entwine them again in the opposite direction. Repeat the steps.
- Unwind your arms. Extend your right arm in front of you, thumb pointing upward. It should be relaxed, not stiff. Place the palm of your left hand behind the elbow and pull your arm to the left as far as it will comfortably go. This stretches the back of the deltoid muscle as well as the outer edges of the trapezius.
- Repeat the stretch on the opposite side.
- Over your clothing, rake your nails lightly over the trapezius muscles, only for a half minute or so. This is a mild version of a technique used by acupuncturists to increase circulation in the surface of the muscle.
- Still working over your clothing, inhale and bring your thumbs up above your clavicles, placing them above the inner edges of the bone. Exhaling, use the pad of your thumb with gentle pressure to stroke from the inside of the clavicle outward. You'll work across sinewy or stringy-feeling cords in the neck called scalenes. Don't use too much pressure on this delicate area. Repeat these outward strokes about ten times.
- Inhale and lean your head sideways to the right. Exhaling, use your left thumb and forefinger to gently grasp the center of the now-relaxed sternocleidomastoid muscle, which feels like a thick cord that runs the length of

the neck, along its side. Roll it gently between your thumb and forefinger, being careful not to pinch, then release it and raise your head. Repeat on the opposite side.

• Inhaling, reach over your head with your right hand until your palm lies flat on the left side of your head, just above the ear. Very gently bend your head toward your right shoulder, exhaling as you do. Release. Do the same on the opposite side. Alternate three sets of stretches, being very mindful of your breathing throughout.

• Remain standing for a moment and bring your awareness to these freshly nourished, well-stretched muscles. The influx of blood (perceptible as warmth) is remarkable. This simple ritual helps ensure that these neglected muscles receive vital nourishment.

AUTUMN SKIN CARE

Our skin is the mirror of our inner health, and, like the rest of our body, is affected by what we eat. Because autumn brings a new focus on respiration, the "third lung," our skin, is also highlighted. Two major influences affect our skin during this time of year. First is dryness, which begins now and continues into the winter. Second is autumn's hormone surge, which is part of our yearly reproductive cycle. In skins prone to acne, this can lead to a period of eruptions and clogged pores that lasts for about a month. This ritual will help you to mitigate the effects of a drier environment.

As we've discussed, whenever a change of en-ergy direction occurs, as it does in the fall, we find air energy, which is always associated with change. Autumn's ruling earth element has a natural affinity for the inner realms of our body, where energy will be concentrated for the lean months ahead. As this nourishing life energy moves inside, the body attempts to preserve stores of fat, and it does not excrete oil as freely as it did in the summer. Oil glands slow their production as the weather cools, allowing dry autumn air to dehydrate the outermost layers of the skin.

Of course, nature's plan is that we increase our consumption of essential fatty acids from nuts and seeds, many of which are harvested now, to ensure that we have adequate amounts of this natural lubricant. In our era of low-fat and no-fat diets, this vital source of nutrition is often neglected altogether.

Women in their mid-thirties will begin to notice the changes brought about by a decline in estrogen production, something made more noticeable when the weather becomes drier. As our skin loses estrogen, it becomes more coarse, affecting its appearance and feel. Recent studies have shown that the estrogenlike isoflavones found in soybeans help keep the skin of premenopausal and menopausal women soft and smooth—as well as protect against some types of cancer. Remember, your skin is a reflection of what's going on inside you—these nutrients are key to keeping your entire body healthy. While essential fatty acids are vital to lustrous, soft skin, they also support proper thyroid and adrenal activity and play a key role in immunity. They have received much attention recently for their ability to promote healthy blood and arteries and for their role in transporting and breaking down cholesterol. On the most basic level, a diet poor in EFAs will leave you vulnerable to the wear and tear of stress and the winter flu season.

If you're experiencing dull, dry skin, this is an excellent treatment you can give yourself. Heat is very therapeutic and helps to stimulate the sebaceous glands, one reason we're oilier in the summertime.

YOU WILL NEED:

A double boiler

1 tablespoon best quality wheat germ oil for topical use
(in the cosmetic section of your natural foods store)

1 fresh avocado, peeled, seeded, and mashed

2 capsules evening primrose oil

3 drops carrot seed oil

3 drops rose absolute essential oil

3 drops sandalwood essential oil

A small bowl for mixing the mask, pre-warmed

A small, clean, soft-bristled basting brush

3 cotton hand towels, one of which you don't care about,

that have not been washed with fabric softener or bleach

Nonalcoholic toner

Moisturizer

• Bring water in lower half of the double boiler to a simmer. Combine the avocado and the oils, stirring gently until warm but not hot. Don't use a microwave, which alters the subtle properties of your ingredients. Transfer to a bowl that you've warmed.

• To freshly cleansed skin, apply the mask, using gentle strokes of the basting brush.

• Fold the three hand towels lengthwise and roll into a tube. Turning each towel end-up, run hot water into the center of the tube, thoroughly wetting the towel. Carefully squeeze out excess, using caution not to scald yourself. Unrolling one towel, let it cool for a moment to bring it to a comfortable temperature. Keep the other towels rolled up tightly. You will use them after the first has cooled down.

• Lie down or recline and place the center of the folded towel at your chin, wrapping the ends up and across your face from both sides, leaving your nose and mouth uncovered. The heat will enable the active ingredients in the mask to better penetrate the skin. Leave the wrap on just until it begins to cool, then replace with the other towel. Repeat once more. You should keep the mask on for ten to fifteen minutes. If time permits, longer is better.

• Remove the wrap, wiping the mixture off your skin with the towel. Be very gentle because towels tend to be more coarse than facecloths. Rinse your face with warm water, then apply a mild, nonalcoholic toner and an appropriate rich moisturizer. We formulated a Hydrating Creme (see Resources) with a base of shea butter, a nourishing natural emollient that's particularly helpful during dry seasons. Shea butter contains allantoin, which has soothing properties and often relieves even severe, itchy dry skin conditions.

AUTUMN SKIN-NOURISHING SNACK

Supplementing the diet with omega-3 fatty acids is an excellent way to ensure that your skin (and your entire body) stays healthy. These fatty acids are found in abundance in flax seed oil and even hemp seed oil. Oil of evening primrose, rich in gamma linoleic acid, can be taken in capsule form. It helps to maintain the skin's softness and flexibility in part by normalizing the behavior of female hormones and is recommended highly for menopausal and perimenopausal conditions, including dry, coarse skin. It is also effective against premenstrual syndrome, including the skin eruptions that typically occur during this time. GLA from evening primrose will restore strength and flexibility to brittle nails and add shine to the hair. Our cosmetic chemist believes in its topical benefits and incorporates evening primrose oil in many of our skin-care formulations.

Because nut and seed oils rancidify very easily, purchase only very fresh cold-pressed organic oils found in the refrigerated section of the natural foods store's supplement department and use them quickly. Rancid oils contain staggering amounts of free radicals and are thought by many health professionals to be highly carcinogenic. Perhaps the best way to enjoy the benefits of nut and seed oils is to eat the whole food. When purchasing seeds and nuts, make sure they are freshly shelled. Buy small amounts and refrigerate them.

Other beneficial oils to include in your skin-beautifying diet are unrefined extra virgin olive oil, sesame oil, and clarified butter, known as ghee and a key ingredient in Ayurvedic remedies.

Here's a recipe for an autumn skin-beautifying snack. Focus on the nutritional value, not the caloric cost. Remember, a small amount is ideal. This mixture is great sprinkled over a salad as well.

YOU WILL NEED:

$^1/_8$ cup freshly roasted pumpkin seeds
$^1/_8$ cup freshly roasted sunflower seeds
$^1/_8$ cup toasted unsalted soybeans (available in bulk
at your natural foods market)
$^1/_4$ cup organic golden raisins
$^1/_4$ cup organic dried pears, chopped
A dash of cayenne pepper (optional)

Combine all ingredients and enjoy. Store in an airtight container, refrigerated. Allow it to come back to room temperature before eating. Make only small batches and use quickly. This is a great midafternoon snack during the day, giving you a protein boost instead of a short-lived carbo "high."

Deep-Cleansing Autumn Acne Treatment

Autumn, the human mating season, treats us to a blast of hormonal excitement. This doesn't manifest itself only in an increased sexual drive. It can create testiness and moodiness as well as serious skin problems. Many of my clients were surprised to discover that they experienced a yearly bout of acne even if their skin didn't normally erupt. Most never remembered that it happened at about the same time each year, so were not prepared for the cycle. If you have noticed that autumn wreaks havoc on your skin, this is a good skin-care ritual to perform.

YOU WILL NEED:

A small bowl

$1/8$ cup kaolin clay (available from a pharmacy)

2 tablespoons organic honey

Tea tree essential oil

Grapefruit essential oil

Fennel essential oil

A small cup

$1/4$ teaspoon of baking soda

2 cotton hand towels that have not been washed with

fabric softener or bleach

• In a small bowl, blend together the kaolin clay and some warm water until you have a smooth paste. Add honey and essential oils. Set aside.

• In a small cup, combine baking soda with $1/4$ cup water. Set aside.

• Cleanse your face twice with a mild, nondrying cleanser. Lightly massage over the skin (minimize any massage if you have active acne) but do not rinse after the second application of cleanser. (Be very careful that you don't get cleanser in your eyes during the next step. If you have two sinks in your home spa, prepare your steaming-sink first.)

• Fill a sink with steaming hot water and add two drops of tea tree oil, two drops of grapefruit oil, and two drops of fennel oil.

• Steam your skin over a sink filled with hot water, allowing the cleanser to remain on the skin for about a minute. Cleansers are purgatives by design. They actually produce a mild "irritation" of the skin in order to flush out the sebaceous glands. This is how cleansers "deep cleanse" the skin, since they do not penetrate into any but the most enlarged of pores.

• Now empty the sink and rinse the skin with warm water. Do not use hot water if you have active eruptions—remember, acne is an *inflammation* and heat will aggravate it.

• Apply your mask thickly to the skin. The clay will effect a purge of the pores. Leave it on for about fifteen minutes. The honey is a humectant that will help keep the mask from getting too hard and dry. Remoisten with a warm, damp towel if the mask is getting dry and cracked.

• Fold a hand towel lengthwise and roll into a tube. Turning the towel end-up, run hot water into the center of the tube, thoroughly wetting the towel. Add a couple of drops of tea tree oil and squeeze the towel a few times to ensure that the essence saturates throughout. Though you still need to use extreme caution when working with hot water, this trick enables you to create a nice steamy towel without scalding your hands. Unrolling the towel, let it cool for a moment to bring it to a comfortable temperature.

• Lie down or recline and place the center of the folded towel at your chin, wrapping the ends up and across your face from both sides, leaving your nose and mouth uncovered. Take a few deep inhalations and enjoy the aromatic properties of tea tree oil. Leave the wrap on just until it begins to cool.

• Remove the wrap, wiping the mixture off your skin with the towel. Be very gentle because towels tend to be more coarse than facecloths. Rinse your face with warm water. Now take a look in the mirror. Sebaceous deposits will be very visible in the openings of the pores.

• The next step is a special massage designed to empty the sebaceous glands. Wash your hands thoroughly with hot water and antibacterial soap. Your skin should now be just dry to the touch. Using your thumb and the broad side of your forefinger, gently grasp the skin of the face, rolling it between your fingers. Do not rub the skin. Work briskly over the entire face, rolling and pinching fingerfuls of skin, for just a few minutes.

• Stir the baking soda/water mixture to mix evenly. Now take a fresh cotton pad moistened with the solution and wipe the skin thoroughly with it. This is called a *disincrustation solution* and it softens follicular debris by making the skin more alkaline (the opposite of its natural pH). Use mild but firm pressure. The cotton fibers will exfoliate the skin lightly and wipe debris from the mouths of the follicles.

• This next step will enable you to remove a visible impaction from the pore. Wrap your middle fingers in a soft, thick layer of cotton saturated in the dis incrustation solution. If you have long fingernails, do not perform this step. When you find a clogged pore, look at the direction that the minute facial hairs grow in that area of the face. This indicates the angle of the follicle in the skin. If you want to cleanse a follicle of debris, you have to coax it toward the opening of the pore. Placing your fingertips alongside a clogged pore, parallel to the growth direction of the follicle, move them back and forth while keeping them parallel to each another. *Use very little pressure. Do not squeeze and do not push inward on the follicle, or it may rupture and cause scarring.* This technique is the only safe way to extract debris from the skin. If you have to resort to pressure, leave the extraction for a professional esthetician. Most estheticians discourage their clients from doing what we call "home surgery." Most of us are not gentle enough. This technique will enable you to cleanse an obvious, visible impaction from the follicle safely. *If you have inflamed pustules, it is imperative that you leave extractions to a medical or skin-care professional to prevent permanent damage and scarring.*

• Saturate a clean cotton pad in toner and wipe over the face for its mild antiseptic benefits.

• Apply an appropriate protection cream or gel. Even oily skin needs to be protected from dehydration. We developed an aromatherapy gel, our Botanical Balancer, for oil-sensitive skin. It contains tea tree oil and viola tricolor to help acne conditions, as well as salicylic acid to help keep the inner surfaces of the follicles exfoliated and free of congestion. We also created a lightweight Clarifying Creme for congested skins that need moisturizing benefits (see Resources).

THE WEEPING RITUAL

In Chinese medicine, autumn is the final display of the earth's richness, and its departure leaves the world saddened. The emotions of the season, grief and worry, suggest a directional change rather than a negative quality in this fascinating season. You may experience an ineffable sadness, or perhaps even a touch of seasonal depression. In Chinese medicine, the sound of autumn is weeping. To a westerner, this may sound unpleasant and a little depressing. Yet being attuned to the season means being comfortable with the changes of nature, not opposing them. Rather than put up resistance to these unsettling emotions, allow your curiosity to lead you on a journey.

This ritual encourages introspection, an inward exploration. The season of outward exploration has ended, and it is time to delve into our interior selves. It is a ritual that allows you to become reacquainted with yin energy, after summer's driving and extroverted yang influence. Whether or not it elicits tears is unimportant. There is no reason to force any sort of response. The key is to simply open the heart. The sound of the season is the voice that echoes inside you.

The use of visualization (sight) and inner dialogue (sound) together is an extraordinary healing blend. Journaling, too, has been documented to speed the emotional healing process. The following exercise utilizes all three modalities. It can be used for a general Body-Mind wellness check-in or to address a specific problem or concern.

YOU WILL NEED:

A quiet, comfortable, and private place where you will
not be interrupted
3 drops rose absolute essential oil
4 drops cedarwood essential oil
4 drops neroli essential oil
An unscented body lotion designed for aromatherapy
blending (see Resources)
A journal, or paper to write on, and a pen

• Get comfortable. It's best to perform this ritual lying down, but you can be gently reclined in a cozy chair. Wear loose-fitting clothing or pajamas. Put a blanket over yourself if you tend to become chilled when lying still.

• Close your eyes and bring your awareness to your breath. Inhale on a slow count of three, and exhale on a count of six, focusing on filling and emptying your entire lung from top to bottom. Feel yourself begin to relax. Do this six times.

• Envision yourself in a place where you feel perfectly safe and at ease. It may be a place of incredible natural beauty, such as a favorite vacation spot. Take a few minutes to create a complete image of this special place. What time of day is it? You may imagine yourself suffused in the glow of a sunset, or enjoying a pale blue dawn. What temperature is the air? Do you feel a soft breeze on your skin, or smell aromatic plants or exotic flowers?

• While you enjoy the feeling of being in this safe, beautiful haven, begin checking in with your entire body, beginning at your feet. Inhale on the same count of three, bringing your attention to the soles of your feet, then exhale for six counts. Focus on your toes, ankles, calves, knees, and thighs in the same way. Silently greet and acknowledge these various parts as you check in. Work your way up, focusing on your buttocks, pelvis, lower back, belly, solar plexus, midback, chest, upper back.

• Move to your fingers and work upward, focusing your attention on your wrists, forearms, elbows, upper arms, shoulders, neck, jaw, cheeks, eyes, forehead, and scalp. This part of the process demonstrates your respect and appreciation for your body and your willingness to listen to it.

• If you have any current conditions that are troubling you, allow your attention to move now to that place. For example, if you've been experiencing low back pain, regardless of whether you currently feel it, imagine yourself visiting the site of the discomfort. If you've had problems with headaches, move your focus to the place where the pain typically appears. Continue to breathe in the same pattern as you do.

• If you've been experiencing emotional upset or stress rather than physical pain, imagine moving into the center of your body and making contact with that emotion. What do you see when you go to this place? Sometimes you'll envision a particular color. An area of pain may appear an angry, brilliant red. Another might be a dull, dead black.

• Make sure that you are in a receptive, open state and then begin a courteous and respectful dialogue with your body: "Is there anything you'd like to tell me?" You may be surprised at the response. For those of us who ignore or discount our bodies' distress signals, this may be the one moment we are really paying respectful attention. Questions posed this way almost always elicit answers.

Other questions can include:

Is there something I should know about you?
Why have I been experiencing this (mental or physical condition)?
What can I do to relieve this (mental or physical condition)?

• As you receive responses from the Body-Mind, try your best to engage in a dialogue. Your inner voice can be startlingly frank and opinionated. It may offer specific advice and direction. It may be gentle and quiet, filling you with a sense of calm and well-being. It will often be filled with emotion, which can create an intense release and outpouring. Whatever the emotional response, allow it to happen. If you feel like crying, allow the tears to flow. It feels wonderful when you are able to relieve the tightness and constriction you sense around the heart chakra. Complete and heartfelt emotional expression is perfectly safe and very healing in such a controlled environment.

• Resist any urge to judge or evaluate what takes place. Instead, when you are finished with the dialogue, slowly bring yourself back. Before you open your eyes, gently tighten and release your muscles from head to toe. Open your eyes slowly and enjoy the sensation of unity you have created between Body and Mind.

• To complete the ritual, take a warm bath or shower to symbolically cleanse the Body-Mind.

• After you pat your skin dry, blend your essential oils into a half ounce of unscented body lotion. Gently massage the aromatic lotion over your entire body. Rose, neroli, and cedarwood are particularly good for healing the heart and releasing sadness or grief.

• To ensure that you benefit from the lessons of your inner wisdom, write down your experience in the journal. Use this as a tangible reminder of your healing journey. Revisit it often and record the progress you make.

• Repeat this ritual as often as needed to promote optimum wellness and cleanse the heart.

WINTER:

SEASON

OF

STILLNESS

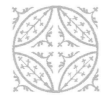

Winter invites us to rest from the frantic activity of the other seasons and to reflect on what we have accomplished. This is the season of sleep for the earth and many of its creatures, and it is the season of stillness and rest for us. It is the end of the earth's fertile period, a time when we focus energy inward, allowing for the replenishment that is vital to future growth. Relations between yin and yang reached their peak in the season of the heart, summer, and came to fruition with the peak of earth energy in autumn, when our fertility was greatest. Now these energies part ways. We may feel a desire to close ourselves off, or we may notice others "cooling" to us. As yang energy declines, we don't feel as strong, generous, or ambitious. We experience the urge to conserve and store.

If you're like many busy people, you may resist the inevitable slowing of winter. You may feel dull and depressed by it, or anxious and irritated because you want to keep moving. When the cold, rain, or snow keeps you inside or affects your commute, your workout, and your daily life, you may feel downright desperate. Even though the weather is doing its best to dampen the fire energy that compels us to get things done, we may still push ourselves to go running in a rain suit or forging across the countryside in snowshoes. And as much as we purport to dislike the madness of the holidays, the stillness that follows can be a little unsettling.

Not surprisingly, the emotion of the season in Eastern medicine is fear. Is it any wonder that we spend more time sick during the winter? On the positive side, fear protects us at the time we're most vulnerable. This is not the time to be bold and take risks. It makes perfect sense to show a healthy fear of the winter world, which can be harsh and unpleasant. But more than that, the ancient fear we experience in winter is that this dark, cold, quiet season won't end. This discomfort with emptiness and stillness is the same one that causes restlessness in meditation and even prevents us from beginning to meditate in the first place. Most of us are used to defining ourselves by the impact we have on our environment, the trail we make as we pass through. Activity is how we feel real and valuable.

Without activity, who are we? This is the perfect season to find out. Winter is the time to let our tracks fill with snow, softening and blurring until our passage is quietly obscured. It's the time to take a deep breath and sit back by a comforting fire. It's time to let someone else take the lead. The rituals of winter will enable you to rediscover your yin side: the gentle art of being receptive and yielding. This is nearly unheard of in our yang-dominated "action" culture. We like to think that we're in control of the events in our lives and believe that taking action is key to success.

But now the seasons of activity and productivity have passed. We don't need to exert our will or express ourselves in the same way we do in the earlier seasons, where our creativity and work are giving shape to our intentions. Thank your squirrel energy for doing such a great job with the nuts, and get yourself some well-deserved rest!

Winter is the season of the feminine. In Chinese medicine, yin is associated with water. Yin energy is at high tide during the winter. In most regions, there is rain or snow. The sound of water can be tremendously soothing, like the gentle patter of rain on the roof. It is a time to observe; our energy shifts inward, our intuition is awakened. It is a season to study, a period in which we are perfectly aligned to absorb nutrition, enjoy quiet companionship, and rest—free of guilt. And yes, we *are* actually designed to put on a few pounds each winter as we store physical energy to see us through the cold season.

The water element that infuses winter rules the emotions. Like water, emotions are changeable and easily diverted, yet possess the power to move mountains. The female body is an eloquent expression of the water element. The movement of water in the body, like the tide, ebbs and flows. We retain water or become dehydrated if we are out of balance. The very same imbalance creates emotional changeability, usually described as moodiness. It can trigger a sudden downpour of tears or an unexpected, snappish reply to a child's innocent question. Water is the element at work when we are experiencing PMS or the mood swings of menopause. The stereotype of the "fickle" woman arises from our susceptibility to the fluid, ever-changing water element. The connection between water and emotion is very real for us. The key to balance during winter is to listen to our inner voice. Our seemingly mysterious mood changes usually occur when we ignore our intuitive wisdom, especially warnings to slow down and pace ourselves. Rituals that acknowledge our inner voice can keep us in harmony with the water element, restoring emotional equilibrium.

During winter, the presence and absence of water are both important themes in self-care. Winter is the season of wetness *and* dryness. Water is no longer evenly distributed through the natural world but concentrated in rain or snow. Water's changeable nature may bring us a deluge one week and painfully dry air the next. During this time, warmth and moisture are needed to comfort and soothe the body. The retreat of life energy from the skin, which begins in autumn, intensifies during the winter. As skin grows drier, it becomes more irritable and easily sensitized. We'll discuss ways to bring the skin into balance during this most challenging season of the year.

THE SOUND FAST

The dense stillness of winter is the hush of a sleeping world. Life is hidden below the surface and we're drawn inward, where life is vibrant. The warm, bright celebrations of the season stave off the quiet only so long. January arrives and we face an emptiness all the more empty for what preceded it!

This simple ritual encourages us to court silence, something that few of us do consciously. Actually, we do nearly everything we can to ensure that silence is eliminated. But this is really our pattern with all the senses: We fill every hour of the day with activity, overwhelming our eyes with an unending stream of images and printed information. We overstimulate our taste buds, and our sense of smell is bombarded with unnatural, engineered fragrances. Our sense of hearing becomes saturated as we consume noise, music, talk radio, and voice mail and fill workdays with meetings.

This ritual is designed to provide relief for your sense of hearing. It is exquisitely simple but harder than it sounds. Your assignment: to find silence and immerse yourself in it. The longer you can do the Sound Fast, the more benefit you'll receive from it.

Vows of silence are an important part of life in many monastic retreats. Silence is one of the essential elements of well-being and necessary for true reflection.

Just as we fast to purify our bodies, a Sound Fast helps to purify our minds. Quieting a chattering mind is possible only when you can create an oasis of actual silence, as you do when you meditate.

• Find a spot where you'll be able to experience at least two hours of uninterrupted silence. It may be in your home, but you might have to venture out to a library or church sanctuary. Expect some unavoidable ambient noise, like the sound of ocean waves, wind in the trees, or traffic in the distance. However, you may get lucky and find a place where the stillness is complete.

• Begin with a simple meditation to create inner quiet. Find a comfortable place to sit and close your eyes. Inhale through your nose on a count of three, filling your lungs from top to bottom. Make sure you feel your belly expand at the end of the inhalation. Exhale through your nose on a count of six.

• Repeat this breathing pattern as you bring your attention to your feet and lower legs. Tense the muscles in this area as hard as you can as you inhale and then try to relax them fully as you exhale. Repeat the 3/6 breath pattern once more, enjoying the relaxation you feel in the muscles, then move to your knees and upper legs, repeating the process. Continue with your gluteals, and then your stomach, chest, shoulders, and arms. Next, tense and release the muscles of the neck, and conclude with the muscles of the scalp and face.

• When you have completed the relaxation sequence, try to maintain the deep, relaxed breathing pattern. Now envision a beautiful crystal-blue light flooding your mind's eye. Imagine it spreading to fill totally your field of vision.

• As you picture this crystal-blue hue, imagine that any sounds you are still hearing are gradually fading away, as if a volume-control knob were being steadily turned down. Tell yourself "The world has become virtually silent."

• Relax for a few minutes, still breathing slowly and deeply.

• Gradually open your eyes. You're ready to begin your Sound Fast.

• During your Sound Fast, engage in any quiet, solitary activity you choose.

Contemplate the landscape, watch the winter sky, paint, or sketch. You can also write in a journal, read something that inspires a sense of peace, meditate, or pray. Don't read the newspaper. You don't have to remain perfectly still, but it's best for the activities to be subdued and low key rather than invigorating, like exercising. If you find yourself resisting this idea, remember that the urge to "layer" activities probably signifies imbalance.

• If you can, try to spend one full day alone this season in complete silence. You'll be delighted at how calm, refreshed, and focused you feel afterward.

WINTER SLEEP ELIXIR

Winter is the season of sleep, when many of the earth's creatures and plants lie slumbering until spring. While humans don't need to hibernate, our bodies are programmed to slow down, rest, and conserve energy at this time of year. Peaceful sleep is essential to seasonal Body-Mind balance. Without its restorative powers, both Body and Mind will cease functioning.

REM sleep is the period in which your brain is sorting, filing, and prioritizing information. As you sleep, neural pathways are being formed between new and stored information, enabling you to access and make use of it. We experience our most intense periods of REM sleep between two A.M. and six A.M.—if we've gone to bed at a reasonable hour and if we're not getting up too early. Though your brain is periodically capable of "making up" for lost REM time, if you maintain a sleep deficit, you will invariably begin to experience serious imbalance, which can lead to problems such as depression, nervous fatigue, or anxiety. Even if the deficit is not severe, your performance and concentration will suffer at work, you won't learn as effectively, and your energy level will be low.

Though many people believe they can "learn" to live with less sleep, without it, the body can't efficiently detoxify its tissues and maintain good health. If you don't get enough sleep, chances are that you're not going to bed early enough. Do you notice that you sometimes feel quite sleepy between nine and ten P.M. and then suddenly get a "second wind" and decide to stay up? You can then remain alert until one or two A.M., when you finally begin to get tired again. You may even feel you do your best work during this quiet time.

If you've had this experience, you experienced the change from earth to fire time. In Eastern thought, the day has cycles that are governed by the different energies—just like the seasons of the year. The energies enable us to be successful at the activities that should be taking place during that time. For example, going to bed with earth energy helps us to fall asleep easily. Earth has a sedating, grounding, and relaxing property.

But fire is the can-do energy that makes things happen. During the night, this energy helps us digest our evening meal. Fire energy can help us through difficult situations where we must remain awake—tending a fussy baby or sick child, dealing with an emergency—because fire provides us with determination and energy. Fire's passion also fuels dancing or lovemaking into the wee hours. Unfortunately, by the time fire rules the night, you've probably missed your chance for sound sleep. You'll probably notice that it's difficult to turn off your thoughts when you do go to bed. If you suffer from fire-induced insomnia, you may find yourself cleaning house or answering e-mail at three o'clock in the morning.

For the most peaceful sleep, it's important to catch the wave of grounding earth energy, which runs from six P.M. to ten P.M. (Remember, these cycles came along long before electricity.) The best time to go to bed is between nine-thirty and ten-thirty P.M. Falling asleep while still riding earth's gentle wave helps encourage sound sleep. It also ensures that you can get up reasonably early and experience a full series of REM sleep cycles. Rising between five-thirty and six-thirty A.M. also ensures that you are aligned with the energy of the day. This enables you to be ready for lunch, which should be your heaviest meal, at around noon to one P.M., when your digestive fires are high. Often, because lunches on the go are rushed and unsatisfying, we find ourselves ravenous at the end of the day and tend to overeat. This in turn creates insomnia. Try not to eat dinner within three hours of going to bed. Eating between six and seven P.M. is best, giving you plenty of time to begin digestion before going to sleep. Avoid caffeine and sugar with your evening meal. More than one glass of wine or beer with your meal will disturb your optimum sleep cycle.

It's also important to exercise awareness when choosing your evening activities. As you get closer to bedtime, lower the intensity level. If you've got work to do, make sure you give yourself at least an hour to relax and release work-related thoughts before bedtime. Stay away from news and television shows that make you feel angry, tense, or anxious. The late news is not bedtime viewing that contributes to sound sleep. Envision your night's rest as a sacred, healing journey that follows very specific stages, each one vital to your well-being. Preparing for sleep mindfully ensures more complete rest and rejuvenation.

The following ritual will help to ease insomnia and encourage sound sleep.

• Drink a cup of calming tea, such as chamomile, to warm, relax, and unwind. There is a marvelous profusion of sleep-enhancing teas at your natural foods store. Bulk teas, sold by the pound, are often more fresh and potent than ones in teabags. Try several and find one you really enjoy. Try not to sweeten your tea, even with honey.

• Enjoy your sleep elixir about ninety minutes before you plan to go to bed. Don't consume liquids within an hour or so of bedtime. Getting up to use the bathroom will detract from the quality of your sleep.

• When you get into bed, place a pillow lengthwise over your stomach and chest. Follow the simple breathwork ritual that begins the Sound Fast. The gentle weight of the pillow helps remind you to expand both your chest and belly as you breathe. It can also serve to ground and calm you if you find it hard to shut off your mind and drift off. (All resemblance to a teddy bear is purely coincidental.)

• If you're getting an adequate amount of sleep, it will take fifteen to twenty minutes for you to drift off. Falling asleep immediately upon getting into bed is simply a sign of sleep deprivation.

RESANCTIFY YOUR BEDROOM

Creating a sacred space for sleep can be a challenge. We tend to think of sleep as a necessary evil. Many of us wish we could use that time for something we believe is more productive. One of the problems in our information-obsessed culture is that our bedrooms have turned into ersatz offices or living rooms. We bring work to bed, use our laptops, or watch news before we fall asleep. It is important that your Body–Mind recognize the bedroom as a place to relax and to sleep. Most Ayurvedic practitioners don't advise doing anything when you get into bed except turning off the light. Even reading in bed is discouraged.

Make sure your bedroom environment is clean, serene, and uncluttered. Take care to tend it as a sacred space. Though you may love having pets sleep with you, their activity will very likely impact the quality of your sleep. You don't even have to be awakened by a pet's nocturnal movements to have your sleep disturbed and its restorative power degraded.

• Make sure that the temperature of your room is not too warm. A bedroom that is a bit on the cool side is much more conducive to sound sleep, and a drop in air temperature is actually one of the "cues" that will help you sleep.
• A slightly open window to supply fresh air will help most people sleep more soundly.

• A cool-mist humidifier is another cold-weather, high-mountain and desert staple. Few of us can sleep peacefully with dried-out nasal passages.

• A mattress that offers proper support and firmness is essential. Your mattress should be turned regularly.

• A pillow that provides the proper support for your head and cervical vertebrae is nearly as important as a good mattress. A "smart foam" pillow that conforms to your head and neck will help ease stiffness and pain in your entire upper body and even reduce muscle-tension headaches. A good pillow helps control restlessness and ensures sound sleep.

ALTAR TO SOUND SLEEP

Your bedside table is the perfect location for a simple altar to sleep.

• Remove any unnecessary clutter from the surface and clean it completely.

• Create a potpourri of fresh juniper or evergreen needles, fresh bay leaves, cinnamon bark, rose hips (which look like little apples in the wintertime), and dried rose petals. The ingredients that you can't gather yourself can be found at an herb store. Place your mixture in a small decorative bowl on your bedside table. A gleaming silver or blue glass bowl is ideal.

• A tabletop or reading lamp that you can dim helps you become sleepy. Bright light will keep you awake; turn off any overhead lights. Candles provide beautiful warm light but can be dangerous if you fall asleep with them still burning. I don't recommend them for this purpose.

• Include a handsomely framed photograph, painting, or sketch of a place that creates a feeling of serenity—a favorite vacation haunt, or somewhere you'd like to visit. It doesn't even need to be real, but this image should evoke a sense of freedom and happiness.

• Refresh and rearrange all the elements of your altar to sleep frequently. Don't let them become dusty, stale, or "invisible."

Sleep-Enhancing Scents

Since earth energy helps you slow down and relax, aromatherapy extracts that increase earth's influence are ideal for a bedtime blend. All aromatherapy extracts are antibacterial and many have antiviral properties, so your immune system will especially benefit from this ritual during a time of year when it's frequently under attack. Be sure to create your sweet sleep blend at night, when you're most attuned to the state of relaxation you're trying to create.

• When creating a blend for sound sleep, remember that your nose knows. First, visualize yourself sleeping peacefully. Take a few deep breaths. Then, using your "personal apothecary" of aromatherapy oils, inhale and note how each oil makes you feel. Narrow down your choices to three essential oils. The oils for enhancing sweet sleep are:

Roman chamomile

Tangerine

Lavender

Clary sage

Jasmine absolute

Neroli

Bergamot

Cinnamon bark

Cypress

• Referring to pages 25 to 30, create a simple blend of no more than three oils that make you feel relaxed. Using three to six drops of each oil (controlling the result by using more or less of each) apply your blend to a cotton handkerchief and slip it into your pillowcase.

• Create a sleep-enhancing room-and-linen spray by combining your three chosen oils, in proportions determined by your nose, in two ounces of distilled water. Put this in an amber or cobalt glass spray bottle, shake well, and spray lightly around your bedroom. Plastic spray pumps will be broken down by essential oils, so you'll need to have a couple of replacements handy.

• It's important to reblend once a week to ensure you have the perfect combination. As conditions in your Body-Mind shift and change, so will your perception of the essential oils.

CLEANSING YOURSELF *of* CARES

I find that bathing at day's end is an important ritual to wash away the "residue" of the day's activities, stress, and cares. A ritual cleansing with hot water at the end of the day can help us achieve a more restful sleep. Sleep-enhancing aromatherapy extracts can be incorporated in a bath oil, a shower gel, or into a lotion or oil used to massage your skin afterward.

For a shower: To two tablespoons of unscented shower gel formulated for aromatherapy blending, add four drops each of lavender, roman chamomile, and tangerine essential oil. Unscented shower gels contain no fragrances or ingredients that can interact with essential oils to create irritation. You can substitute rose absolute for the tangerine oil if you like. It's particularly beneficial if you are feeling disheartened, discouraged, or even a little unloved.

Work the blended gel into a net sponge to create a lather and bathe luxuriously. The steam of the shower is a terrific aid to inhalation of essential oils.

For a bath: In a small glass bottle, add two drops each of lavender, tangerine, and roman chamomile essential oil to one tablespoon squalane or jojoba oil. Shake it vigorously and add to your bathwater as your tub is filling. Dim the lights or light a candle, which will help you become sleepy. Be careful that your bath is not too hot; it will be overstimulating and may keep you awake.

BEDTIME SELF-MASSAGE

When the weather is dry and cold, and when you are under stress, you may be prone to racing thoughts and excessive nervous energy. If you are traveling a lot by air, you may become "ungrounded" and overly anxious. Even a fast elevator ride in a high-rise building can be unbalancing, leaving you dizzy and even a little disoriented. Insomnia is often a sign of excess air energy, which keeps the mind active.

Ayurvedic practitioners long ago discovered that self-massage using generous amounts of oil could reduce nervousness and anxiety. Combining aromatherapy with oiling is particularly beneficial for keeping you healthy during the wintertime. Daily use of essential oils is believed to create a higher level of resistance to illness by stimulating the activity of white blood cells. A noted aromatherapist, whose essential oils we use at the spa, tells a story of having a blood test by a physician who was stunned by the activity of her white blood cells. The doctor was so impressed by the incredible aggression of her white blood cells toward pathogens seen under the microscope that she demanded to know what she was doing. The aromatherapist explained that she worked with essential oils and used them daily.

A favorite choice of our clients for this ritual is the Warming Ginger Massage Oil we use at Preston Wynne (see Resources), made with an organic extract of ginger and some of the spices used in the recipe below. It's comforting and rich and smells just heavenly—the perfect oil for winter body care. Cinnamon essential oil is especially known for its effectiveness against viruses.

⁓ *Bedtime Massage Recipe* ⁓

❋

Caution: Cinnamon is a strong oil that should not be used undiluted on the skin. Do not use this blend on your face or before sun exposure!

To three tablespoons of organic sesame oil (found at
the natural foods store) add any three of the following essential oils:
2 to 3 drops mandarin orange
1 to 2 drops cinnamon leaf
2 to 3 drops roman chamomile
1 to 3 drops clary sage
You can use less of any of the oils if you wish.

• Make sure the bathroom or area you're using for your massage is warm, cozy, and private. Play some soft, relaxing music and dim the lights if possible.

• Seat yourself on a stool, chair, or the edge of your bathtub on a towel. This treatment can get a little messy, so be prepared for drips.

• Be generous with your oiling—the quantity is important. The sensation should be luxurious.

• Start by closing your eyes, then inhaling deeply for three counts. Exhale for six counts. Pausing between each inhalation and exhalation, repeat three times before beginning your massage.

FACE SEQUENCE

Caution: Do not massage the face if you have an active acne condition. You can warm the oil you'll be using by immersing its container in some hot water, or you can warm the oil in the beaker of a small coffeemaker. You'll need only a teaspoon or so for the facial massage. Add three drops of roman chamomile and three drops of mandarin orange essential oil. These are soothing oils and they smell quite wonderful together; they have a relaxing effect on the nervous system as well, which makes them a perfect remedy for insomnia.

- Interlace the fingers of the hands and lay them over the forehead. Stroke outward, pulling the hands very slowly apart. Repeat this six times. Quick massage is stimulating, not relaxing. A slow stroke with medium pressure is very soothing to the nervous system.
- Circle back around the orbit of the eye, stroking from the temple toward the nose underneath the eye with light pressure. This is delicate skin; don't stretch it. When you come to the center, use thumb pressure on the point just below the browbone on the inside corner of your eye. If you have a lot of muscle tension there, or if you have headaches frequently, this may hurt. Press up, as if you're lifting the browbone. Repeat at least three times.
- Grasp the heavy corrugator (brow) muscle between your thumb and forefinger, rolling and pinching it gently.
- Place your thumbs under the cheekbones where they begin alongside the nose. Press upward from under the bone, gently rotating in a barely perceptible circle for six seconds. Work your way outward. You will have about five pressure points.

• At the outside of the cheekbone, drop down about a finger's width and press your middle finger on the powerful muscle that operates your jaw. Open your mouth slightly and press into the muscle, using a slight circular movement to give variation in pressure.

• Pressing the pads of your fingers into the temples, rotate slowly using medium pressure.

SCALP SEQUENCE

The muscles of the head are usually very tight and this is an area that is easy to work on yourself. The jojoba oil is good for emulsifying and softening sebum deposits in the skin and on the scalp.

• Using your fingertips, massage the scalp as if you were washing your hair.

• Then press your fingertips flat against your scalp and without moving them over the skin, shift the scalp forward and backward, working from the temples to the top of the head.

• Placing your hands on the sides of the head, rub your thumbs over the occipital ridge at the base of the skull. Do this once while sitting up straight and facing forward. Then slowly roll your head back and repeat. Keeping your hands in the same position, work your thumbs into the hollows under the ears. Push your thumbs from the outside of the skull back toward the center, then from the inside outward.

• Once again, with fingertips pressed to the scalp, move the scalp in small, circular motions. Finish this step by pressing on the soft depressions in the temples, forming almost imperceptible circles, for about six breaths.

• Gently grasp your hair with both hands and pull slowly, but not so much that your scalp hurts. Some scalps are very sensitive.

BODY SEQUENCE

• Rest your foot on your leg and apply oil to the bottom and top; squeeze the sides of the foot to "fold" it over. Massage gently but firmly, pressing with your thumbs into the arch of the foot. Cross your leg at the knee and let the foot drop so you can see the top of it. Gently push the toes down to stretch the shin. "Clean between the tendons" of the feet, working down toward the toes. Holding the foot in one hand, gently grasp and pull on each toe with the other hand.

• Apply oil generously to the legs, working up the calves and shins with a hand-over-hand stroke toward the heart. "Wring" the lower leg between your hands.

• Massage the upper legs, always working toward the heart.

• Oil the arms and work upward from the wrist. Always begin with light strokes before working more deeply.

• Work the hands. Use moderate thumb pressure to work the muscles in the palm of the hand to the ends of the fingers, then squeeze the sides to "fold" the hand. Finish by pulling on the fingers gently.

• Conclude by lightly running your hands over your entire body with sweeping movements. Slowly sweep down the legs and off the feet—a quick sweep is energizing. Sweep down the arms and off the hands. Envision yourself sweeping off the cares and stress of the day, exhaling through your mouth by making a soft "shhuhh!" sound as you do.

• When you're done, take a shower and cleanse thoroughly.

Caution: Launder oil-saturated towels thoroughly, using the pre-soak cycle, hot water, and extra detergent. Oil residue in towels can create a fire hazard.

TAKING BACK
the LIGHT

During the winter, you'll probably find yourself with less energy than usual. Many men and women experience symptoms of what is known as seasonal affective disorder, an imbalance or depression linked to reduced exposure to ultraviolet light. The reduced light of winter is compounded by the fact that we're indoors more to avoid inclement weather. A poorly lit environment can intensify conditions of sensory deprivation. In the office, artificial lighting from fluorescent fixtures offers only a portion of the wavelengths of light your brain needs to remain healthy. While it's been proven that introducing an additional source of ultraviolet light can be helpful, SAD is a limited explanation for a more complex seasonal response by the Body–Mind. Your energy has moved inward in response to cues from the natural world, which include a reduction in ultraviolet light as well as dropping temperatures. Your metabolism has slowed to assist you in keeping weight on for warmth and energy storage. Your activity level has diminished, as has your interest in interacting with others. Water's influence creates a reflective state that brings you into touch with your emotions and feelings. These forces all work together to produce the most introverted state you'll experience during the year.

Here are some simple practices that will help you "lighten up."

• Open your curtains and drapes as much as possible during the day.

• If possible, change the bulbs in fluorescent fixtures to ones that incorporate a wider range of the light spectrum. These are available from any commercial lighting supplier. Ask for full spectrum bulbs.

• Get up with the sunrise. If possible, take a walk, but don't engage in a strenuous workout, which can deplete you further. Breathing deeply during your walk helps to enhance the flow of lymph through your body, detoxifying your tissues and restoring energy.

• When outdoors, minimize the amount of time that you wear sunglasses, allowing your eyes to receive the full spectrum of light wavelengths. In the wintertime, wear sunglasses for safety only.

THE GODDESS FEAST

Culturing and nurturing our friendships is a key element of self-care and another important aspect of life that often falls to the wayside amid our busy schedules. Friendships require time and attention, but they will usually take a backseat to other more urgent activities.

The Goddess Feast is a special ritual for midwinter that celebrates friendship between women during the season that encompasses the pinnacle of yin's feminine energy. This is a great way to relax after the hubbub of the holidays, a season that is often filled with obligatory and less enjoyable rituals. With the pressure off to shop and prepare for family gatherings, we can explore this quiet season of reflection in the company of good friends.

This ritual is designed to nurture you on several levels. First, there is a simple and comforting midwinter feast to prepare and enjoy together. By gathering in the kitchen—the "heart of the home"—we open ourselves to nourishment and love. Second, this ritual is designed to nurture you with friendship. In past generations, the pooled efforts of the community or tribe were necessary to ensure survival through this, the harshest season. Winter is naturally a time to be with other people, another reason that the holidays can be difficult for a person who does not have a network of friends or family. Third, this ritual is designed to honor and celebrate feminine energy and feminine strength.

Winter is the natural season for what we've come to call "comfort food." These richer, denser, tissue-building foods are designed to help build strength and internal heat. They also increase our body weight for the long winter—a natural phenomenon that is often complicated by the high consumption of sugar and fat that takes place during the holidays.

Since water energy rules the season, we may experience it in excess—a condition known in Chinese medicine as "dampness." We can be left feeling lethargic and depressed, or showing symptoms of edema or excessive weight gain. To counteract dampness, eat warming foods that increase fire's influence. The hearty soups of winter are perfect for this. Roots are where the energy of plants is concentrated right now, so root vegetables are particularly attuning in the winter diet. Roasted beets, parsnips, turnips, carrots, onions, and potatoes are traditional staples of winter cooking, and these humble root vegetables have enjoyed a revival with the rise of New American cuisine. Roasting them with some olive oil and a bit of sea salt enables the flavors to concentrate and deepen. Roasting is the perfect cooking method for winter, when it's better to reduce the amount of water and increase the amount of time we use in cooking. Roasting imbues food with fire energy, something that can help ensure we remain warm enough.

Sun-dried fruits, in small amounts, help to offset the water energy of wintertime; their water content has been dried up by the sun. Imbued with fire energy, they bring a ray of summer sunshine to the winter diet. Fruits that are harvested in the fall are more attuning, including raisins, apples, and pears. Use them sparingly, because they have high concentrations of sugar. Dried tomatoes, currants, and cranberries are wonderful complements to savory dishes as well.

Even if out-of-season produce is widely available, try as much as you can to eat foods in season, such as root vegetables, winter greens, legumes, and seeds. Eating lots of fresh fruit or raw vegetables in the wintertime creates excess water energy and can cause you to feel cold and weak. Keep your food combinations simple to facilitate easy digestion. This is important especially if you have animal protein in your diet. The following ritual includes recipes that can be part of any balancing wintertime meal.

Allow time for you and your friends to prepare the dishes in your Goddess Feast together rather than having one person act as a hostess or chef. The foods in the feast are rich, warming, and hearty, the very essence of comfort food. Fat is used moderately but without apology! Even though this is a vegetarian menu, it's far from boring, and it's the perfect foil for a light red wine such as a Côtes du Rhône.

Every flavor of the taste spectrum is represented, especially the underused bitter flavor, which is found in the spinach, endive, pear skin, and some of the vegetables.

Savory Bread Pudding with Roasted Winter Vegetables

This humble, hearty dish is the essence of comfort food and the perfect main dish for a cold winter evening. It utilizes roasted winter vegetables to create a warming meal that is full of rich, concentrated flavors.

3 tablespoons extra virgin olive oil

1 yellow onion

Choose winter vegetables, organic if available, such as beets, turnips, parsnips, winter squash, carrots, celery root, eggplant, and portobello mushrooms.

2 teaspoons sea salt

Pepper to taste

1¹/₃ cups organic low-fat milk

2 eggs

4 slices stale sourdough bread

4 slices stale whole grain bread

$^1/_4$ cup grated Reggiano cheese

$^1/_4$ cup crumbled fresh goat cheese

1. Preheat oven to 375 degrees.

2. Rub a baking sheet with extra virgin olive oil. Cut onion and as-sorted vegetables into chunky pieces, leaving the root vegetables whole. Drizzle with a generous amount of olive oil and arrange on baking sheet. Sprinkle with two teaspoons of sea salt, which will extract water and con-centrate the flavors. Roast the vegetables for at least 30 minutes, removing them as they finish cooking and setting them aside until all are thorough-ly cooked. They will brown and shrivel—don't worry about their appear-ance. They'll taste wonderful. Roast the onion until it has virtually caramelized.

3. After allowing them to cool enough to handle safely, slip the skins off the root vegetables and chop them into chunks. Pepper to taste.

4. Increase oven temperature to 400 degrees. Butter a two-quart bak-ing dish.

Whisk together the milk and eggs. Tear up the breads and saturate pieces with the milk/egg mixture, covering the bottom of the baking dish with them. Put a layer of vegetables over this and sprinkle with a mixture of the cheeses. Add another layer of bread, another layer of vegetables, and pour the remaining egg/milk mixture over all. Top with the remaining cheese.

5. Bake about 20 minutes, finishing with a minute under the broiler to brown the cheese.

Warm Salad of Spinach, Endive, and Pear with Pine Nuts and Parmesan

The sweetness of the pear, balsamic vinegar, and pine nuts is a lovely contrast to the bitterness of the endive, spinach, and the peel of the pear.

¹/₃ cup pine nuts

3 cups tender baby spinach leaves, washed and dried

2 tablespoons balsamic vinegar

¹/₃ cup olive oil

1 cup endive leaves, cut into 1-inch pieces

1 crisp but ripe winter pear (Comice, Anjou) washed but not peeled

¹/₄ cup Parmesan, thinly shaved into approximately 1-inch pieces

Salt and freshly ground pepper

1. Place pine nuts on a baking sheet and toast, shaking the pan several times to turn them, for 4 minutes at 350 degrees. Remove to a paper towel until needed.

2. Toss the spinach, vinegar, and pine nuts in a bowl.

3. Heat the olive oil almost to the point of smoking. Pour it over the spinach and pine nuts and toss until all the leaves are coated and wilted.

4. Add the endive, pear, and cheese and gently toss until they're also coated with the dressing, taking care not to break them up. You may need to add a bit more vinegar. Add salt and pepper to taste.

Baby Carrot-Ginger Soup with Mint Crème Fraîche

2 tablespoons chopped fresh mint

$^1/_2$ cup crème fraîche

4 tablespoons butter or ghee

4 shallots, chopped

$^1/_2$ cup red wine

2 tablespoons grated fresh ginger

Juice of half a lemon

$2^1/_2$ pounds washed organic baby carrots, diced

$7^1/_2$ cups vegetarian "chicken" stock (available at natural foods stores)

2 pinches cayenne pepper

Salt and pepper

1. Dice the mint finely. Gently fold it into crème fraiche and allow to stand at room temperature while you prepare the soup. This gives the plant's oils time to pervade the crème fraîche.

2. Melt the butter or ghee in a soup pot. Add shallots and cook for five minutes. Add the wine and ginger and cook until most of the liquid is absorbed, about 3 to 5 minutes, being careful not to let it burn.

3. Deglaze the kettle with the lemon juice, then add the carrots, stock, and cayenne and bring to a boil. Reduce heat and cover, simmering until the carrots are tender, about 35 minutes.

4. Let soup cool enough to puree in a blender or food processor. Return to the kettle and heat. Season to taste. Serve with a generous dollop of the mint crème fraîche.

Winter Fruit Poached in Zinfandel

Juice and zest of 1 lemon (Meyer lemon if available)
1 cup of very good quality California zinfandel, such as Ravenswood
or Peachy Canyon
2 tablespoons pure organic maple syrup
Dried figs, apples, and pears
1 cup organic whipping cream, room temperature
Nutmeg
Biscotti

1. Zest the lemon with a peeler, then chop finely, reserving a few long peels for garnish.

2. In a saucepan, heat wine, lemon juice, maple syrup, and half the zest until boiling. Add dried fruit to the mixture and reduce to a simmer. Simmer for 20 minutes, then allow to stand for 10 more.

3. Whip cream lightly, adding a small amount of nutmeg. Spoon a small amount over the warm fruit and garnish with a pinch of lemon zest, a dash of nutmeg, and some crunchy little biscotti.

THE TOASTING RITUAL

Celebrating our accomplishments is something we usually do privately and discreetly. And celebrating our inherent beauty is something we may not do at all. This ritual calls for a suspension of any and all self-deprecating language that women use to talk about ourselves.

• Set the mood for this ritual with some vintage vocal jazz by the greats: Ella Fitzgerald, Sarah Vaughan, Billie Holiday, Betty Carter, or Carmen Mac-Rae.

• You'll need a few simple supplies: some elegant paper such as a fine stationery or parchment paper, a pen with metallic gold ink, and a ten-inch piece of blue ribbon for each guest. In Chinese medicine, dark blue is the color of winter, but more important, a blue ribbon is a symbol of reward and triumph.

• Propose a toast to another member of the group. Describe something that she recently accomplished, a unique but little-known talent she possesses, a heroic act of friendship, her extraordinary beauty, graciousness, or intelligence. Go around the table until everyone has been acknowledged at least once; let it continue—it probably will.

• Now that you're all warmed up and in a magnanimous mood, here's the hard part! Each woman must now propose a toast to herself, extolling her intelligence, beauty, or romantic prowess, and professional, athletic, or artistic successes. Any woman who lapses into self-deprecation, even in humor, must start her speech all over again! This speech must continue until even the shyest member of the group has declared her charms to the world in unequivocal terms.

• While this is happening, a "scribe" will record each declaration on the paper, roll it up, and tie it with a blue ribbon to be given to the guest as a souvenir and affirmation.

Make your Goddess Feast a winter tradition every year.

WINTER SKIN
SURVIVAL

Winter's harsh weather can be the undoing of any skin type—even one that's not normally given to problems with dryness. The skin's sensitivity increases with dryness, and even a familiar moisturizer, when used to treat chapped, wind-burned, or severely dry skin, can feel irritating rather than soothing. This two-step emergency treatment is designed to help your skin recover from overexposure to the elements. In the first phase, you'll hydrate and soothe the skin, initiating the healing process. The antioxidants in the green tea and the soothing agents in the chamomile will help calm the skin. In the second phase, you'll seal the skin with protective, nourishing emollients to prevent loss of moisture.

YOU WILL NEED.

2 tablespoons pure, cold-pressed aloe vera gel

(available from your natural foods store)

¹/₄ cup loose chamomile tea

A pinch of best-quality jasmine (green) tea, preferably

jasmine pearl

2 capsules evening primrose oil

¹/₂ teaspoon hemp seed oil (available at your natural foods

store in the personal-care department)

3 pieces pure cotton batting (available at any drugstore) cut into

4-inch-long strips (the batting sheets are about 10 inches across)

1 shallow one-quart bowl

1 hand towel

1 small natural sponge

• Prepare a comfortable place to lie down with your treatment mask on, and place the towel over a pillow. Have a blanket handy for warmth.

• Brew the chamomile and green tea and allow it to steep for fifteen minutes. The tea should be dark amber gold in color.

• Strain the tea leaves and pour tea into the bowl to cool to room temperature.

• Immerse the pieces of cotton batting and the natural sponge in the tea and allow them to become saturated.

• Secure your hair with a band or towel and gently cleanse your skin with your usual cleanser. Rinse well with tepid water and pat dry.

• Apply the aloe vera gel generously with your fingers. Don't be concerned if the aloe vera makes your face turn slightly pink. (This is not normally a sign of allergic reaction, though there are some individuals who are allergic to aloe vera.)

• Now, squeeze excess moisture from one of the pieces of cotton batting, but make sure it is still well saturated. Mold it gently over your forehead. Take the second piece and mold it over the lower face, leaving the nose and mouth free. Mold the third piece over the center of the face. Lie down, but take the moistened sponge with you to add more of the tea solution to the mask once you are horizontal. It may drip a bit, so the towel is useful.

• Relax with your compress mask on for at least fifteen minutes, preferably twenty. Make sure to cover yourself with the blanket so that you don't become chilled.

• Remove the compresses and discard. Blend the evening primrose and hemp seed oils in the palms of your hands, allowing your hands to warm them a bit.

• *Important: If you have active acne, skip this step completely and apply additional aloe vera gel instead.* Massage the nourishing oils over the entire face, using slow, gentle, upward strokes. If your skin is irritated, minimize massage manipulations.

• Use gentle pressure with your fingertips on the inside corners of the nose, pulsing and rotating your fingers slightly without lifting them. Hold, pulsing gently for six seconds, then release. Place your three center fingers on your temples and do the same. Now move under the cheekbones on the sides of the face, applying the same gentle pressure for six seconds. Move back toward the jaw muscle and repeat. Staying just under the ridge of the cheekbone, do the same for the front of the face. Repeat this series two to three times. These pressure-point massage manipulations are helpful for opening the sinuses, which are also affected by harsh, cold weather. Remember, your respiratory system and your skin are interconnected. Your sinuses can contribute to red, blotchy, or sensitized skin if they become inflamed or congested.

TIPS FOR PREVENTING WINTER DRYNESS

• Don't assume that your summertime moisturizer is going to work. For some people, it does. But most women find that they need to supplement their everyday moisturizer during the winter or use a richer formula altogether.

• Try this test to see if your cleanser is too drying for wintertime use. Wash your face but don't apply moisturizer for two minutes afterward. If your face feels taut and dry immediately after cleansing, consider switching to a milky or creamy cleanser. All skin types should use a cleanser that's free of stripping detergent ingredients but is still capable of emulsifying oils and makeup.

• Make sure you always use a nonalcoholic toner during the winter, unless your skin is still extremely oily. Very few people need to use a toner that contains alcohol. Instead, your toner should contain moisture-attracting humectants such as sodium PCA and glycerin. We developed our Botanical Freshener, which contains essential oils like lemongrass, lavender, and geranium, as an all-skin-type balancing toner (see Resources). Toner should be used to restore pH after water is used to rinse the skin. The pH of water is alkaline, making it especially drying to the skin during the wintertime.

• Certain types of exfoliating cosmeceuticals like alpha hydroxy acid, retinol, or retinoic acid may prove to be more drying to your skin during the winter. You may need to reduce your frequency of use to achieve a comfortable balance.

• Drinking enough water is important, but also important is the water in the air around you. A cool-mist humidifier is an important addition to your bedroom in the wintertime.

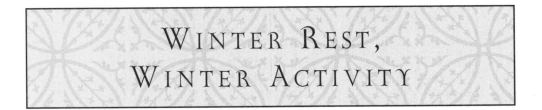

WINTER REST, WINTER ACTIVITY

Yang energy has gone, and yin's influence means that our mental energies now take precedence over physical energies. Even so, staying active is important to keeping the Body-Mind in balance. Yoga is tremendously helpful for ensuring that we stay flexible during the cold season and is an excellent way to keep life energy flowing freely.

If you're one of the people piling into the gym after the holidays, you have an uphill battle ahead of you! This is a not a season to train hard, and it's a difficult time to begin an ambitious workout program. Your body is not designed for strenuous activity during the winter, but, rather, for conserving energy. Of course, this does not mean that you should become completely sedentary.

Your lymphatic system relies on the movement of the lungs and the muscles to gently pump lymph fluid through the tissues. During the winter flu and cold season, your immune system is repeatedly challenged; keeping the lymph moving ensures that your body is properly detoxifying itself. This is one of the primary benefits of regular physical activity.

For a winter workout, walking is ideal. If you are in a snowy climate, the new lightweight, easy-to-use snowshoes can keep you moving throughout the season. Despite the fact that you should be avoiding cold, damp conditions in excess, your Body-Mind becomes attuned to the season when you go outdoors and stimulate your senses with the unique sights, sounds, smells, tastes, and textures of winter. Dress appropriately for winter workouts. Exercise gear that wicks perspiration away from the skin is very important to prevent becoming chilled.

WINTER BODY BRUSHING WORKOUT

Body brushing, or dry brushing, is a detoxifying treatment for the body's "third lung," the skin. Like exercise, body brushing stimulates the flow of lymph and blood, cleansing the tissues of waste and clarifying our thinking. Dry brushing even provides gentle cardiovascular conditioning; in fact, it has been used for cardiovascular exercise in the space program. When you try this body-brushing "workout," you'll be surprised at how it elevates your heart rate. It can be a wonderful exercise alternative when the weather is bad—or when *you're* feeling under the weather. Body brushing is an excellent way to begin a gray, gloomy winter day in a brighter mood.

Always wash your brushes after using them with a mild soap and dry them, bristles down, on a clean towel. This prevents water from seeping into the brush head and damaging the wood and bristles.

Caution: Do not perform this ritual if you have any inflammation, open wounds, or skin eruptions. Do not perform if you have been diagnosed with or are being treated for cancer. If you are pregnant, consult your health-care practitioner before dry brushing.

YOU WILL NEED:

A good-quality vegetable-bristle body brush with a
wooden handle (available at natural foods stores, in the
personal care section, or see Resources)
A natural-bristle nailbrush
A natural-bristle foot brush
A warm, comfortable treatment area with good
air circulation
3 drops lavender essential oil
6 drops eucalyptus essential oil

• Disrobe completely for your dry-brushing workout.

• Put three drops of lavender essential oil on the palm of your hand and lightly apply it to the bristles of the dry brush.

• Be mindful of your breath as you do your dry-brushing workout. Exhale smoothly as you complete the long strokes just as you would when performing an exercise. Inhale using relaxed but deep breaths.

UPPER BODY SEQUENCE

• Begin with very light pressure. You can increase it gradually, but the benefits of dry brushing are accomplished with fairly light but firm pressure. Raise your left arm over your head and brush the underarm area using five clockwise circular strokes. Then perform five counterclockwise circular strokes. This provides gentle stimulation for the lymph nodes. Repeat with the right arm, switching your brush to the other hand. You can grasp the brush by the head rather than the handle for more control.

• With your arm still elevated, brush upward from the top of the breast, working outward toward the underarm. Be careful to avoid the breasts, which are too delicate for dry brushing. Work from the center of the sternum outward, using overlapping strokes, then raise your opposite arm and repeat the sequence in the other direction.

• Place the brush on the breastbone and brush up and around the right breast, stroking outward toward the left underarm five times. Now complete five strokes using your left hand, working from the center around the breast toward the left underarm area.

• Now place your brush on your left side at the waist and stroke upward under the arm. Do this five times. Use sweeping, even stroke pressure, exhaling as you do. Repeat on the right side.

• Now reach over your shoulder to place your dry brush on the spine, at the inside edge of your right shoulder blade. Stroke outward toward the right shoulder five times. Here the handle of the brush will give you needed leverage. Repeat on the left side, completing five strokes.

• With the brush now in your left hand, place it on the back of your neck. Sweep it down and around the neck toward the collarbone. Repeat this five times on the left side, then switch hands and repeat the stroke on the right side. Be careful when working around the neck, as this skin is very delicate and sensitive. Using lighter pressure, brush along the neck under the left jaw, then sweep the brush down the sides and to the collarbone. Perform just three repetitions. Complete the sequence once more on the right side for three repetitions.

• Place the brush gently under the chin and brush down the neck to the collarbone with very light pressure. Repeat just three times.

SCALP AND HEAD SEQUENCE

• Place your dry brush at the nape of the neck and sweep it up over the back of the head toward the forehead. Typically, a bit more pressure is comfortable on the scalp. Repeat eight to ten times. Brushing relaxes the muscles of the scalp and can be very enjoyable. It also stimulates blood circulation to the hair follicles, helping to ensure healthy hair and scalp.

• Now grasp the brush by the head and move it over the scalp in circular movements until you have completely massaged and brushed the entire scalp. To complete the lymph drainage, brush downward from the top of the head, stopping at the ears. Repeat this stroke five times.

HAND AND ARM SEQUENCE

Note: Complete this entire sequence on the left side before moving to the right hand and arm.

• Using the small nailbrush, work back and forth across the nails and cuticles with light but firm pressure. Turn your hands over and massage the brush over the palms from the fingertips toward the wrists.

• Switch to the large brush and stroke from the fingernails toward the elbow on the top of the arm. Repeat six times, then repeat the sequence from the palm to the elbow on the underside of the arm. The underside is quite delicate, so you'll need to use lighter pressure here.

• Now use the brush on the upper arm, stroking from the elbow to the shoulder six times.

ABDOMINAL SEQUENCE

• Place your brush at the top of the left hipbone. Stroke seven times down toward the pubic area. Never brush the genitals. The groin is a major lymph drainage point. Repeat on the right side.

• Place the brush next to the navel and brush in clockwise circles over the abdomen seven times.

• Place the brush under the left breast and stroke down to the groin three times. Repeat on the right side.

BACK SEQUENCE

• Holding your brush in your right hand, place it on the tailbone. Brush outward over the right buttock and then around toward the groin. Begin once more at the center, and lowering the brush, work down over the entire buttock, repeating the sequence until you reach the top of the leg. Now complete the sequence on the left side.

• With your brush in your right hand, complete seven strokes up the center of the back. Follow with seven strokes on the right side of the back, switch hands, and finish with seven strokes on the left side. You can use firm pressure on the back; it feels wonderful. You should also notice by now that your respiration and pulse have markedly increased.

FOOT AND LEG SEQUENCE

• Using your foot brush, massage the soles of the feet with firm circular strokes. This helps to exfoliate the feet and it stimulates the many nerve endings there. If you're not ticklish, you'll enjoy the sensation. Spend a minute brushing the feet if you can. Use your nailbrush to brush the nail and cuticles of the toes, then switch back to the large body brush to brush the feet from the toes toward the ankles. Repeat seven upward strokes on each side.

• The lower legs are a common area for water retention. Dry brushing can help alleviate this condition. Place the brush near the ankle and stroke firmly upward toward the knees. Work your way around the leg. Repeat on each side twelve times, more if you have puffiness around the ankles.

• If you have puffiness around the knees, this sequence will be helpful. Place your brush just below the knee, on the front of the leg. Brush back around the knee. Your target are the lymph nodes behind the knees. Repeat seven times on each side.

Note: Complete the full thigh sequence on each leg before moving to the opposite side.

• The thighs are an area full of lymphatic vessels and prone to congestion and stagnation. Touch the outer thighs and note the temperature there—it's usually much cooler than other parts of your body. Dry brushing helps to stimulate circulation, which aids in the cleansing and detoxification of these tissues. Place your brush on the inside of the right knee and stroke upward, crossing the front of the thigh, toward the groin. Repeat three times. Begin the next stroke by placing your brush higher on the inner thigh, again stroking across toward the groin. Repeat three times. Work your way up until the stroke is nearly horizontal, repeating each one three times. You can use more pressure for this stroke. It's a good sign if the thighs redden slightly from the stimulation of the brush.

• Place your brush on the right outer knee and stroke upward three times, crossing over the front of the leg toward the groin to complete the stroke.

• Place your brush at the back of the knee and stroke upward toward the buttock three times, using firm pressure. By now you should have brushed the entire upper right leg. Repeat the entire sequence on the left side.

• Now move to the lower leg. The reason we begin with the upper leg is to open the lymph vessels there first, since they are closest to the lymph nodes in the groin. This then allows us to move fluid from the lower legs upward, without blockage. Begin with your brush on the front of the right leg, at the ankle. Brush upward with five strokes, swirling the brush around to finish behind the knee. Move the brush to the right side of the lower leg, just at the ankle. Brush upward again, finishing behind the knee. Move the brush to the left side and use five strokes; finish with the brush behind the knee once more. Repeat the entire sequence on the left side. You should be breathing as you might during a brisk walk.

• If you have time, repeat the upper leg sequence again for a more complete drainage and a more vigorous workout.

• Finish the dry-brushing workout with a warm shower. Sprinkle six drops of eucalyptus essential oil around the edges of the shower and breath deeply. Towel-dry vigorously afterward. You should feel alive and vital from head to toe!

Winter Hibernation

During this season of dreams, you may feel a little drowsier than usual. Your energy has moved inward. As long as your are moderately active and eating a balanced diet, this shouldn't be a problem. But if you're having to wake yourself up with a jarring alarm and a shot of caffeine every morning, you probably need to increase the amount of sleep you're getting.

A nap is a simple and often overlooked rejuvenating ritual. Cultures that enjoy siesta tend to have a healthier approach to other basic daily activities, such as eating. You can derive substantial benefit from a nap of even just ten minutes, but try not to nap for longer than thirty minutes on a regular basis. A nap ritual can even make your workday more productive and less draining, significantly easing stress and enhancing your ability to focus. If possible, taking a brief nap during that energy dip in the afternoon instead of a caffeine-and-sugar infusion can contribute greatly to your overall Mind–Body balance.

- A strong urge to sleep immediately after eating is usually a sign of imbalance and digestive disturbance. In such instances, a brisk ten-minute walk will be more restorative and balancing.
- Find a quiet spot to nap but preferably not your bedroom. Your Mind–Body association to the bed is sleeping, not napping. You need to be comfortable to nap well but not *too* comfortable.
- If you're at work, put your phone on "do not disturb." If you have an office with a door, a polite sign lets others know not to disturb you. Though it's not good for a real nap, you can sit in a chair and put your head down on your desk. If the ergonomics of napping at your desk aren't good, weather permitting you can nap in your car.

• Make sure that you'll stay warm enough. Your body temperature is affected by even a short catnap. A light blanket or throw is fine.

• Before your nap, gently and slowly massage your hands for about two to three minutes with a soothing and aromatic hand balm (or make your own from the recipe that follows). Do this each time you nap and the scent will quickly become a powerful sleep suggestion. Like your feet, your hands are full of reflex points for all your vital organs. However, in the hands these reflex points are much deeper and harder to activate. Of particular interest for your health in the wintertime are the points in the fingertips, which correspond with the sinuses. If you're having colds or sinus problems, you may find them tender when you apply deep pressure.

Soothing Winter Hand Balm

Dry hands and cuticles are a problem for nearly everyone during the winter, and the shea butter in this balm will help ease dryness and irritation. Chamomile is well known for its skin-soothing and relaxing properties. Clary sage is a rich, smoky, and euphoric essence that must be used sparingly if you plan to get any work done after your nap. Jasmine, also a euphoric, is particularly beneficial for the feminine endocrine system, and because of its yin balancing properties is effective against wintertime depression. Lavender helps ensure that all the oils "marry" harmoniously.

4 drops clary sage essential oil
6 drops roman chamomile essential oil
8 drops jasmine absolute essential oil
4 drops lavender essential oil.
¹/₄ cup pure shea butter (available from the natural foods store's
personal-care department)

In a small bowl, mix essential oils and the shea butter together thoroughly with a plastic spatula. The friction created when mixing the butter will warm and melt it slightly, making it easy to incorporate all the essential oils. Store in an airtight glass container, preparing only a small amount at a time to ensure freshness. Label the container with a one-month "expiration" date.

WINTER BRAIN BREAK

A very simple, easy alternative to napping for mental rest in winter is a Brain Break, which can refresh your mind and help restore your focus.

• Turn off the phone or put it on "do not disturb." A cubicle dweller I know puts a sticky note on her back that declares simply "I'm invisible" to discourage visitors.

• Keep some earplugs handy, or a headset with a quiet, relaxing piece of instrumental music to drown out the background buzz of the work environment.

• The key to this ritual is remaining perfectly motionless, except for the steady, smooth motion of your breathing. Once you're comfortably seated in a chair with your hands resting, palms up, in your lap, close your eyes. Do not adjust, shift, or fidget. Sit absolutely still for just five minutes, breathing slowly and evenly through your nose. Allow your awareness to visit areas of discomfort or stiffness, and breathe into the spot to help relax it.

• Open your eyes and enjoy a surprising feeling of refreshment.

This is a simple technique that can help even the most distracted and preoccupied person begin a meditation too. By keeping the body motionless, we force the mind to slow down too. Remember, the Body-Mind connection works both ways.

WINTER REVIVING MEDITATION

It's not always possible for us to slow our lives down with the arrival of winter. At work and at home, adapting our daily routines to a more gentle pace can be difficult. When we persist in maintaining a demanding schedule, imbalance can result. Though sometimes this seasonal imbalance takes the form of colds or flu, it may also be experienced as exhaustion or a feeling of depletion.

This reviving meditation can help restore mental and physical energy. I was first introduced to it by Robert Sachs, an expert in Tibetan Ayurveda. I recommend his book, *Health for Life*, as an excellent guide to well-being through Tibetan Ayurvedic practices. (See Resources.)

- Sit on the floor or in a comfortable chair. If seated on the floor cross-legged, fold a towel or place a small cushion beneath your tailbone to allow your knees to be below the level of your navel. Rest your hands, palms down, on the tops of your legs.
- Instead of closing your eyes completely, gaze downward at the floor just beyond your knees, following the line of your nose. If you are seated in a chair, you can look between your knees at the floor.
- Inhale slowly through the nose and then contract your stomach, groin, and

buttocks. Hold your breath briefly, then exhale, feeling yourself relaxing into the cushion beneath you.

• Focus your awareness on the breath entering and exiting your nostrils. Feel your abdomen expand easily with inhalations as you draw air in through the nose. Experience the movement of the air through the nose. As you exhale, direct the breath toward the area on the floor your eyes are gently focused on. Imagine your breath melting away at this point.

• Anytime your attention strays from your breath, gently redirect your focus back to it. Breathe at a natural, easy pace.

• After you have been doing this for about five minutes, you can add a mantra to help balance the energy of the root chakra and reconnect your Body-Mind to the earth. Silently repeat the sound *lum* to yourself with each exhalation. Continue this for about ten more minutes. This primordial sound is used in Ayurvedic meditation because of its unique resonance with earth energy. If your attention wanders, gently bring it back to the mantra. Mantras are useful for helping us maintain proper focus in meditation and preventing the intrusion of mundane thoughts. More important, mantras also have a particular resonance with a different energy center of the body. Mantras have no literal meaning. The sound's vibration produces its benefit to our consciousness.

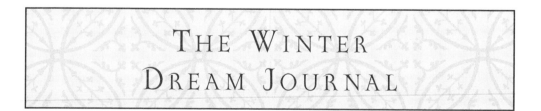

THE WINTER DREAM JOURNAL

Winter gives us an opportunity to reflect on the previous seasons and assimilate the lessons of our year. Much of this work may happen on an unconscious level during this season if you align yourself with the receptive, observing energy of winter. This is an excellent time to deepen an existing meditation practice or begin a new one.

As we've discussed, the water element rules winter, heightening intuition and sensitivity. Because we are more receptive during yin season, and because we are less physically active, this is a natural time to pay attention to what's going on in our subconscious. Though winter is an excellent season to begin recording dreams, the practice should continue throughout the seasons of the year. Our dreams can be a key to self-knowledge and greatly inform our personal practice of self-care. Messages about your well-being, life purpose, and relationships bubble up from a hidden well of wisdom and insight. Taking an interest in our dreams is a way that any of us can acknowledge soul in our daily existence. Capturing them is simple.

If you recall, dreaming occurs during our periods of REM sleep. REM sleep occurs in the early morning hours, and our longest REM sleep cycle happens just before we awaken.

- Keep a dream journal beside your bed. It does not have to be an elegant blank book. If it is, you'll be tempted to record only dreams that seem "worthy." Choose something that you are not intimidated to write in, such as a simple lined notebook. This will encourage you to write down everything!
- As you go to bed, tell yourself that you will remember what you dream about. This step is tremendously helpful.
- As soon as you awaken, write down what you remember of your dreams. At first, you may draw a blank. You may be able to recall fragments. But as you make a habit of recording your dreams, you will remember more and more of them.
- Make a memory elixir to keep by your bedside:

10 drops rosemary essential oil
18 drops lavender essential oil

Combine and place in a $1/2$-ounce cobalt or amber glass dropper bottle.

To use, sprinkle a couple of drops on a handkerchief and inhale deeply. Rosemary is considered an aid to memory by herbalists. This practice also creates a subconscious association, ensuring that the fragrance will soon become connected with remembering your dreams. Because all essential oils affect the portion of the brain responsible for memory and bypass the mind's cognitive processes, they can help you more freely explore yin's subconscious dream world.
• After you've written down your dream, read the account aloud. Its meaning is often clarified by this simple act.

Dream interpretation is a strange blend of science and art. Humans seem to have an incredible set of symbols that appear in our dreams, regardless of our culture, our sex, or our age. Some dreams contain messages that turn on words used to describe what is seen or what occurs, often as puns. Some dreams have symbolic and metaphoric messages that are as obvious as billboards. Others appear to be pure nonsense, while some are like an irritating snooze alarm that saves us from oversleeping or in some cases even danger.

Dreams are the adventures of our subtle bodies. Some are mundane—like a trip to the etheric grocery store—and some are profound, like a grueling quest to a secret holy place. Resist the temptation to edit your dreams, no matter how absurd or tedious they may seem at first. Your dream journal should bring the richness of your inner life to your everyday existence, unabridged and without judgment. Dreams contain lessons and messages even when they are woven from a fabric we don't entirely understand.

THE NEW YEAR
VISION WALK

The first day of the year can often be a curious letdown after the hoopla of New Year celebrations. If spending most of the day watching football doesn't feel like the best way to inaugurate the new year, you can try this visualization ritual instead. This is a day of power, a portentous moment. A gorgeous blue sky on New Year's day may tell us that the year ahead is going to be terrific. A heavy sky and sheets of rain may make us question all our plans and dreams.

The key element of the Vision Walk is time: It is meant to be a long walk. A significant element of physical challenge helps to set this apart from other walks you might undertake. It does not have to be grueling, but it needs to be a *journey*. You need to walk long enough to fall into an unconscious rhythm, to experience a state in which the Body-Mind has found a certain accord and harmony, conditions ripe for dreaming while awake. This special day provides you with an opportunity to occupy the moment fully and to carry that experience of awareness with you into the new year. The Vision Walk can be a hugely satisfying ritual of rebirth that you'll look forward to year after year.

- If possible, plan your Vision Walk as a large circle rather than an out-and-back route. The circle symbolizes wholeness and completion. It also symbolizes the center. The Vision Walk may be a journey, but during it you should be truly centered and in the moment.
- The Vision Walk is best as a solitary activity, but if you need to take a companion along for safety reasons, make sure you're both participating in the ritual. You may even agree to maintain silence during the walk, speaking only when necessary to check your route or stop for water.
- Don't hurry. The steady movement of the walk is important. If you are for-

tunate enough to have beautiful scenery to enjoy, all the better, but carefully observing whatever is around you, regardless of its apparent aesthetic value, is more important. If you're truly aware and receptive, you'll find yourself discovering beauty in strange places. The Vision Walk is a walking meditation. Direct your awareness to commonplace details: a particular arrangement of flotsam near a storm drain, the hardware on a gate, the color of rosehips, the texture of clouds, the smell of wet soil, the taste of rain. Stop if there's something you'd like to examine or experience more completely. Envision yourself as a sensory sponge, taking in all that you see, hear, feel, smell, and touch as if you had arrived from another planet. Acknowledge your intuitive yin energy and enjoy the sensory stimuli without analysis. Later you'll have a chance to create a context for what you've experienced.

• You may find a token of your Vision Walk to bring home with you. You can add this small object to an altar and use it to remind yourself of your vision for the year. If you have made commitments to yourself, focusing on this object can help you return to the day of beginnings and refresh your inspiration for change and growth.

• As with a dream, there's no need to press for meaning, but you will usually discover something interesting if you ask. When you return, sit quietly for a moment, for ten to fifteen minutes in meditation. (See the Winter Reviving Meditation pages 224 to 225.)

• When you're finished, write down whatever you remember, even if it seems mundane. This is a new year and your new world. What did you discover when your eyes were open and your attention expanded? What surprised you? What was exquisite? What was painful, sad, or distressing?

This is a personal journey, symbolic of the journey you are undertaking in the new year. Consider if this journey has changed your feelings about the new year or yourself. What have you discovered? What did you see that made a deep impression? What other sensory experiences affected you?

Keep a collection of your New Year's Vision Walk journals. They make for fascinating reading as your life progresses.

RESOURCES

To help you choose the best tools for your seasonal rituals, I've included a list of professional quality spa products that are wonderfully effective, many of which are a part of the Preston Wynne Spa Collection. You should by no means limit yourself to these—there are dozens of excellent products on the market today that are available at natural health and beauty stores as well as salons and spas. This list is intended to help you get started, but feel free to substitute similar products that you prefer. Remember, you are the best judge of which items will work best with your individual seasonal health and beauty needs.

PRODUCTS FROM THE PRESTON WYNNE SPA COLLECTION CAN BE ORDERED BY CALLING 1-(800) 747-5525 OR BY VISITING THE SPA AT WWW.PRESTONWYNNE.COM.

Detoxifying Seawater Bath
    Algae Bath Concentrate, Preston Wynne
    Nourishing Body Moisturizer, Preston Wynne Spa Collection

Spring Exfoliation Treatment
    Fruit Enzyme Peel, Preston Wynne
    Clarifying Sea Mineral Mask, Preston Wynne Spa Collection
    Moisture Creme for Sensitive Skin, Preston Wynne Spa Collection
    Botanical Balancer for Oily and Acneic Skin, Preston Wynne Spa Collection

SUMMER

Summer Tea-Time Ritual
    Jasmine Pearl Tea
    Imperial Tea Court
    1411 Powell St.
    San Francisco, CA 94133
    1-(415) 788-6080

After-Swim Summer Skin Care
    Sea Refresher Bath and Shower Gel, Preston Wynne Spa Collection
    Seaweed Oil for Skin Hydration, Preston Wynne
    Nourishing Body Moisturizer, Preston Wynne Spa Collection
    Ultimate Foot Care Creme, Preston Wynne Spa Collection, Foot Nourisher
    by I/O. Neti pot, New Life Products 1-(800) 852-3082

AUTUMN

Relief for Tired Eyes
Body and Soul Stones are available through Preston Wynne

Anxiety-Easing Mud Treatment
Body Brushing Starter Kit
1-(877) YOUGLOW

After-Work Aromatherapy
Unscented lotion for aromatherapy blending, Aroma Vera

Autumn Skin Care
Hydrating Creme, Preston Wynne Spa Collection

Deep Cleansing Autumn Acne Treatment
Clarifying Creme for Oily Problem Skin, Preston Wynne Spa Collection
Unscented lotion for aromatherapy blending, Aroma Vera

Developing Strength and Routine
For a studio in your area providing instruction in The Method (exercises and equipment of Joseph Pilates)
1-(800) 505-1990

WINTER

Bedtime Self-Massage
Warming Ginger Massage Oil, Preston Wynne

Winter Skin Survival

    Botanical Toner, Preston Wynne Spa Collection

Winter Reviving Meditation

    Health for Life: Secrets of Tibetan Ayurveda by Robert Sachs

    Heartsfire Books

    500 N. Guadalupe St. Suite G-465

    Santa Fe, NM 87501

Winter Body Brushing Workout

    Body Brushing Starter Kit

    1-(877) YOUGLOW

ABOUT PRESTON WYNNE SPA

Preston Wynne Spa in Saratoga, California, was founded as a specialty skin-care salon in 1984 by Peggy Wynne Borgman and Douglas Preston, both estheticians by training. The salon has since evolved into one of the most respected day spas in the country and has twice been named Day Spa of the Year by *Spa Management Journal.* In 1999, Preston Wynne was named Distinguished Day Spa of the Year by the Day Spa Association. Preston Wynne's innovative treatments for the skin and body have attracted a loyal following of clients from all over the San Francisco Bay Area.

In addition to its renowned skin care and body therapy offerings, the spa's menu includes integrative yoga therapy, metabolic nutritional consultation, acupuncture, Chinese herbal medicine, and hypnotherapy. Preston Wynne also features a makeup department with a philosophy that reflects its natural approach to beauty. This diverse palette of treatments and services is drawn upon to create Personal Paths, goal-oriented programs for well-being and personal image that span four to twelve weeks.

Peggy Borgman is the director of Preston Wynne Spa, which has a staff of sixty estheticians, body therapists, and support personnel. Douglas Preston heads the company's consulting division, Preston Wynne Success Systems, which serves the spa and salon industry with education, technical training, professional products, management, and spa startup consulting.

For reservations or information on the spa, please call 1-(408) 741-5525 or send e-mail to dayspa@caprestonwynne.com. Visit the spa's Web site at prestonwynne.com. To contact Preston Wynne Success Systems, call 1-(408) 741-1750, extension 12.

INDEX

peppermint leaves, 124–26
peppermint tea, 99
    in relief for tired eyes,
        138–40
perimenopause, 173
Personal Path, 7–8, 48
petrissage, 96
Pilates, Joseph, 161
Pilates method, 92–93, 160–61
pine essential oil:
    for respiration blend, 153–54
Pitchford, Paul, 108
plants, 41–42
polarity, 58
posture, 90, 91–92
potpourri, for altar to sound
        sleep, 194
prana, 112
pranayama, 110–11
pregnancy, warnings for, 29, 137,
        155, 215
premenstrual syndrome (PMS),
        25, 95, 173, 187
Preston Wynne Spa, 45, 48, 198
Preston Wynne Spa Collection,
        62
pumpkin seeds, in autumn skin-
        nourishing snack, 173–74
purification, 41

quadricep exercise, 164

radicchio, in cooling summer
        chopped salad, 101–2
raisins, 204
    in autumn skin-nourishing
        snack, 173–74
raspberry conserves, in heat
        balancing salsa, 103
raspberry leaf, 99
reawakening the artist, 79–81
red bell pepper:
    in cooling summer chopped
        salad, 101–2
    in simple autumn dinner,
        157–58

in a simple red feast for
        summer, 105–6
reflexology, 34–35, 139
Reike, 58
relief for tired eyes, 137–40
remineralization, 61
removing your armor, 90–93
REM sleep, 190, 191, 226
resanctifying your bedroom,
        193–94
respiration blend, 153–54
retinoic acid, 214
retinol, 49, 71, 214
retreats and rituals, 82–83
rice vinegar, in a simple red feast
        for summer, 105–6
rituals, 2, 8, 12–13, 16, 22, 33
    aromatherapy and, 26–27,
        121–22
    bathing and, 41, 56–58
    body image and, 19–21
    eating and, 45
    exercise and, 47
    facial-care, 72–73
    healing arts and, 19
    intention of, 63
    retreats and, 82–83
    sacred space and, 40
    sound and, 32
    temperature contrast shower,
        36
    touch and, 33
    see also specific seasons
Rolfing, 92
romaine lettuce, in cooling
        summer chopped salad,
        101–2
roman chamomile essential oil:
    in bedtime self-massage,
        197–201
    in cleansing yourself of cares,
        195–96
    as sleep-enhancing scent,
        195–96
    in soothing winter hand
        balm, 222–23
root chakra, 225
root vegetables, 132–33, 204
rose absolute essential oil, 27,
        59

in autumn skin care,
        171–72
    in weeping ritual, 179, 181,
        196–97
rosemary essential oil, 27
    in after-work aromatherapy,
        155–56
    for winter dream journal,
        226–27
roses, 26, 122

Sachs, Robert, 224
sacred space, 11, 40–43, 107,
        147–48, 193–94
    sanctuary for the heart,
        121–22
    summer tea-time ritual and,
        100
    see also altars
salad, chopped, cooling summer,
        101–2
salicylic acid, 178
salmon, in a simple red feast for
        summer, 105–6
salsa, heat balancing, 103
salutation to the sun, 111–14,
        115
sandalwood essential oil, 27, 72,
        73
    in autumn skin care,
        171–72
    in summer sanctuary for the
        heart, 121–22
savory bread pudding with
        roasted winter vegetables,
        205–6
scalp and head sequence, in
        winter body brushing
        workout, 217–18
scalp sequence, in bedtime self-
        massage, 200
sea mineral wraps, 94
seasonal affective disorder (SAD),
        202
seasonal cycles, 1–4, 7–8, 9–13,
        141
    body image and, 20–21
    cooking and, 44–45

music in, 108
sun protection in, 49–50
touch and, 120
visualization and, 39
walking in, 117
water and, 97–98, 119–21
yang energy and, 17, 32, 60, 120, 131
summer healing arts:
after-swim skin care, 118–19
altar to joy, 107–8
body contouring massage, 93–98
morning meditation, 37, 109–11
removing your armor, 90–93
salutation to the sun, 111–14
sanctuary for the heart, 121–22
swimming as, 115–17
summer sensory therapy:
hearing therapy and, 30–32
heat wave tea bath, 124–26
keeping cool with food, 101–6
landscape infusion, 122–24
laughing ritual, 126–28
taste therapy and, 24
tea-time ritual, 98–101
walking barefoot as, 119–21
sunburn, 124
sun-dried fruit, 204
sunflowers, 135–36
sunflower seeds, in autumn skin-nourishing snack, 173–74
sunlight, 88, 202–3
sun protection, 49–50, 69, 109, 116, 119, 203
sunrise, 109
fire element and, 16
in winter, 202
Swedish bodywork, 6, 34
sweet pepper, in a simple red feast for summer, 105–6

Tai Chi, 47
taking back the light, 202–3

tangerine essential oil, 27
as sleep-enhancing scent, 195–96
Taoist philosophy, 14, 78
tapotement, 97
taste, 15, 20
in summer, 10
tea-time ritual and, 100
therapy, 24–25
tea-time ritual, 98–101
tea tree essential oil, 27, 121
in deep-cleansing autumn acne treatment, 175–78
temperature contrasts, bathing and, 36, 57–58
therapeutic touch, 13, 33–35
see also massage
third lung, see skin care
throat chakra, 74, 90, 91
thyme essential oil:
in after-work aromatherapy, 155–56
Tibetan Ayurveda, 137, 224, 225
titanium dioxide, 109
toasting ritual, 210–11
tomato, in a simple red feast for summer, 105–6
toner, 49, 118, 173, 213
touch, 32–36
ki and, 34–35
seasons and, 10–11, 120
swimming and, 116
tea-time ritual and, 100
see also massage
Trager, 34
Transcendental Meditation, 37, 38
transitional seasons, 3, 31, 36, 89, 131–34, 140–41, 145, 147, 152, 153
trapezius, 167, 169
exercise for, 166–67
travel, 12
treatments:
anxiety-easing mud, 140–44
deep-cleansing autumn acne, 175–78
for dry skin, 171–73
see also detoxification therapies; exfoliation

tricep exercises, 166
turnips, 204
in savory bread pudding with roasted winter vegetables, 205–6

upper back exercises, 168–70
upper body exercises, 165
upper body sequence, in winter body brushing workout, 216–17

vanilla essential oil:
for aromatherapy linen mist, 146–47
varicose veins, 137
viola tricolor, 178
vision, see sight
vision for the year ahead, 81–83
visualization, 12, 32, 39–40, 179
body image and, 20
spring and, 69
vitamin A, 150
vitamin C, 49
vitamin D, 46, 108–9
vitamin E, 118

wake-up ritual, 104
walking, 69–70
barefoot, 119–21
New Year vision and, 228–29
in summer, 117, 123–24
in winter, 202–3, 214–15
Warming Ginger Massage Oil, 198
warm salad of spinach, endive, and pear with pine nuts and Parmesan, 207
warm-stone therapy, 7
warm-up, 160
water, 16, 69, 88, 97–98, 214
retention of, 219
water element, 24, 187
balneotherapy and, 36